Curing and Healing

Curing and Healing

Medical Anthropology in Global Perspective

Andrew Strathern
and
Pamela J. Stewart

Department of Anthropology
University of Pittsburgh

Carolina Academic Press
Durham, North Carolina

Library of Congress Cataloging-in-Publication Data

Strathern, Andrew.
    Curing and healing : medical anthropology in global perspective /
Andrew Strathern and Pamela J. Stewart.
      p.   cm.
    Includes bibliographical references.
    ISBN 0-89089-942-8
    1. Medical anthropology. 2. Rites and ceremonies. 3. Healing.
4. Traditional medicine.   I. Stewart, Pamela J.   II. Title.
GN296.S79   1999
306.4'61—dc21   99-13187
                                                  CIP

Cover photograph: Skulls of relatives cared for in a limestone rock ledge at Hagu (Duna, Papua New Guinea). In the recess of the ledge is the cradle-like container made for the remains of a dead child. Picture taken in 1998 (see Ch. 5).

CAROLINA ACADEMIC PRESS
700 Kent Street
Durham, North Carolina 27701
Telephone (919) 489-7486
Fax (919) 493-5668
E-mail: cap@cap-press.com
www.cap-press.com

Printed in the United States of America

Contents

About the Authors

Prof. Andrew Strathern and Dr. Pamela J. Stewart are a husband and wife research team who work in the Highlands (Hagen, Duna, and Pangia areas) of Papua New Guinea and the Lowlands (Ayrshire area) of Scotland.

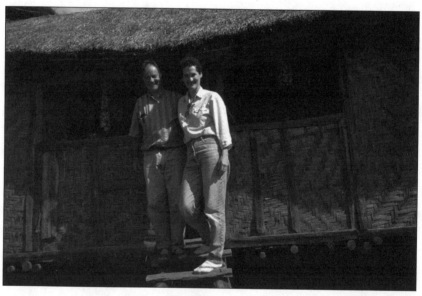

The two fieldworkers at the verandah steps of their house in Hagu among the Duna (1998).

Acknowledgments

We wish to thank Ms. Joan Paluzzi for assistance with the text of Chapter 2 on Latin American ideas and Ms. Leah Voors for help with the questions supplied in conjunction with each chapter. Both were supported through the Dean's fund in the Faculty of Arts and Sciences at the University of Pittsburgh. Fieldwork among the Duna people of Papua New Guinea was supported partly by the Pitcairn-Crabbe Foundation, administered by the Department of Religious Studies at the University of Pittsburgh. Ms. Rachel Chapin-Paolone assisted with the typing of the manuscript. Parts of the manuscript were written while we were based at the Centre for Pacific Studies in the School of Anthropology and Archaeology, James Cook University, Townsville, Australia in mid-1998. The copy-edited text was finally checked while we were Visiting Senior Fellows at the International Institute for Asian Studies, Leiden. We thank all of these institutions for their support, as well as a number of individual colleagues in the Medical Anthropology Discussion Group at the University of Pittsburgh for their interest in our project. Kaja Finkler also gave initial encouragement to proceed with the book. For all shortcomings we remain responsible.

Leiden, The Netherlands
December 1998

Curing and Healing

Chapter One

Introduction

Overview

Medical anthropology is one of the newer subdisciplines of anthropology, itself a relative newcomer in the arena of scientific and humanistic studies. It began with an interest in ethnomedicine: the practices of peoples around the world aimed at dealing with sickness and enhancing health. Accounts of these practices were seen to belong to the broader accounts of social and cultural patterns in which ideas about sickness and health are universally embedded. More recently, medical anthropologists have extended their interests, first to various forms of alternative medicine imported from contexts that were seen as belonging to ethnomedicine, as for example Native American forms of healing that have been incorporated into New Age practices in the United States; and second into the analysis of biomedical practices, those that hold in mainstream medical systems in metropolitan countries.

The movement of medical anthropology has, in fact, been a kind of circular migration: from the jungle to the city, and back again. Completing the circle is important because biomedical practices and institutions have been introduced world-wide and come into relations of accommodation and conflict with local indigenous practices based on very different premises about the human body and the world. These interactions give rise to a situation described as pluralism, in which people make complex choices about forms of treatment derived from both indigenous and introduced notions. This situation is by no means new in human history, but it has been accelerating during the second half of the twentieth century. In the twenty-first century we may see a further global blending of ideas which will mean that versions of pluralism are more readily evident everywhere; or we may not. This book aims to give readers an idea of the complexities of ideas about sickness and treatment regimens with a worldwide focus, considering biomedical and other regimens within the same conspectus of cultural and social analysis. From this perspective, a patient's consultation with a doctor in Europe or America is amenable to analysis just as much

3

as the activities of a healer using indigenous spells and herbal remedies in Amazonia or New Guinea.

Other Introductions

Most subfields of anthropology by now can boast of multiple alternative introductions. There is a whole industry, for example, in producing introductory volumes on cultural or social anthropology in general. In medical anthropology there are also a number of good existing introductory textbooks. By comparing the present work to a few of these we will indicate ways in which our book is different. One of the older standard textbooks is George Foster and Barbara Anderson's *Medical Anthropology* (1978). This is a very well- balanced early survey of the field, particularly useful for its exposition of what it calls the "strengths and weaknesses" of non-Western medical systems, a theme that also concerns us here. Separate parts of the book deal with "the non-Western world" and "the Western World." While this was perhaps a valid and pragmatic way of arranging materials at the time, it is not one we have systematically chosen to follow. The mixing and globalization of ideas and practices and their continuing local transformations in response to such mixing all mean that we need to look at the case materials in a single conspectus, that of contemporary world history. This does not mean that we obliterate, elide, or gloss over differences, since differences between systems give us vital clues to their comparison and explanation. It does mean that we take every opportunity to make plain the connection between local and wider influences on the customs and modes of behavior we discuss. Foster and Anderson in practice also followed this way of thinking. Foster, for example, has argued that the "humoral" ways of thinking in South America (e.g. notions about hot and cold as these affect the body) are a blend of indigenous notions and the principles of ancient Greek medicine (Hippocratic, derived from the fifth century B.C. physician Hippocrates) introduced through the Hispanic conquest from the sixteenth century A.D. onwards (Foster and Anderson 1978:59, Foster 1994). This means that he recognizes that the following centuries have witnessed a blending of "western" and "non-western" features that makes it an option to bring "the west" and "the rest" together rather than separate them, even if for purposes of exposition it may be necessary at times to refer to ideas by their origins in this way.

One of the topics dealt with briefly by Foster and Anderson is medical ecology (1978: 11–32, also ch. 15). Another textbook, by Ann McElroy and Patricia Townsend (1985), goes into this branch of the subject in much greater detail. A feature of their admirable book is that much of it is organized around the concept of adaptation which they define as "changes and modifications that enable a person or group to survive in a given environment" (1985:12). They go on to state that "health is a measure of environmental adaptation" (p. 13), so that health can be studied by an approach through ecology, the ways in which people adjust to, and influence, their environments. This approach stresses the perspective of the outside observer who uses biological models of ecosystems to measure the degree of adaptation achieved by a given population. The approach is valid and illuminating. For instance, by using it we can analyze, as McElroy and Townsend do, Inuit cultural adaptations to Arctic conditions by comparison with the physical adaptations of polar bears that share the same environment. Inuit population densities were kept low when groups still depended largely on hunting; the people wore warm clothing obtained by hunting animals and processing skins; and they ate a diet with a high protein and a low carbohydrate content, including raw meat that gave them vitamin C and bones which yielded calcium, thus achieving a high metabolic rate that helped to keep them warm. By concentrating on diet in this way, the authors are able to draw attention to the adaptive achievements of particular peoples and the risks involved in upsetting these adaptations. We will draw on this perspective as needed, particularly in relation to epidemiological issues. We pay greater attention, however, to the whole range of cultural ideas that people themselves may bring to bear on the conditions of their life, setting their own ideas about the body and health into their wider pictures of the cosmos and their place within it. We also wish to avoid giving a picture that no longer applies. Later in their book McElroy and Townsend show how health conditions of the Inuit declined with sedentarism, diet change, and reservation life, including alcoholism — results of historical forces that overcame their earlier adaptations to the environment. It is important also to remember that adaptation can involve practices that may be seen as harsh from other outside perspectives, for example female infanticide practiced as a means of population control.

A third textbook is Cecil Helman's *Culture, Health and Illness* (3rd ed. 1994), a remarkably well-documented and wide-ranging overview which uses a very large number of case-histories and quantitative citations from all over the world. This book does not attempt to duplicate the range of examples Helman gives. Its goal is to deal with fewer cases in greater detail, and to build on these cases so that they can illuminate more than one theme, for example, medical pluralism as well as ethnomedicine in case materials from Japan (Ohnuki-Tierney 1984), Mexico (Finkler 1994a), and New Guinea (Frankel 1986, Frankel and Lewis 1989). We follow Helman, however, in insisting that medical systems have to be seen in terms of overall theories of, and the experience of, the human body; and that medical processes, such as going into and coming out of hospital, can be seen as forms of ritual just as healing ceremonies around the world have been seen in this light. In other words, Helman's perspective is global, both geographically and analytically, as ours is. However, this book stresses the significance of in-depth ethnographic findings even more than his does. By concentrating on a smaller set of cases, it aims to give readers an impression of what the American anthropologist Clifford Geertz called "thick description" (Geertz 1973) without making the resulting "stew" too unpalatable to swallow.

Concepts

Thick description cannot in fact simply depend on making a stew that appeals to a range of tastes. Its ingredients must include sets of concepts. We use three pairs of concepts that interrelate with each other and are important for our general perspective. These are:

1. The distinction between disease and illness.
2. The distinction between curing and healing (which appears in our title and is the basis for our conclusions (Ch. 14)).
3. The relationship between mind and body.

1. Disease and Illness

Horacio Fabrega (1974) and Arthur Kleinman (1980) have made a useful distinction between these two concepts. Kaja Finkler (1994a:5) renders Kleinman's version of this distinction as follows: "disease is defined as a biological and biochemical malfunction, and illness as impaired functioning as perceived by the patient within the cultural context."

It is important to recognize that if we define the distinction in this way, the concept of disease is one that belongs primarily to biomedicine, i.e. the contemporary form of scientific thinking that prevails regarding medical regimens and which has developed in Europe and America since the eighteenth century. Illness, however, is a concept that is likely to be shared by peoples of many different cultural backgrounds around the world. This disparity of reference puts some limitations on the use of the concepts while suggesting that one of them, illness, is universal or nearly so. Accepting this limitation, we can go on to say that within biomedically dominated contexts physicians are also likely to concentrate on the aspect of disease, while patients are more concerned with the whole experience of being unwell, that is, with their illness. Second, while in some cultures the concept of disease may be lacking in biomedical terms, analogous ideas may be present that enable us to see how people distinguish narrowly between a particular condition and the wider experience of suffering from it and showing its symptoms. In some instances, however, this would lead us to broaden the definition of "disease" too greatly, as when we would refer to an idea of "spirit attack" as a concept of disease. We have to be pragmatic in our usage of the term. At the widest level, though, the distinction is useful in terms of the difference between a narrow definition of a condition (disease) and its broader experiential setting (illness), a distinction that may coincide with a difference of perspective between the "doctor" and the "patient" in a given case.

2. Curing and Healing

This distinction matches to some extent with the first. As we, and other medical anthropologists, use the term, curing refers to an act of treating successfully a specific condition, for example a wound or a case of diarrhea or infestation by worms. Healing, by contrast, refers to the whole person or the whole body seen as an integrated system with both physical and spiritual components. Biomedicine, in this view, deals with curing and not healing; alternative medicine and the medical systems of various cultures may depend on a philosophy of healing that either encompasses or stands outside of curing.

Here also there are some limitations and dangers. In a given cultural context we cannot necessarily expect to find an equal stress on both curing and healing practices. One may also predominate over the other, or the two may be comfortably or uneasily balanced. Practices may be strong in one sphere, less so in others. Foster and Anderson's(1978) evaluation pointed out that "non-Western" systems are often strong in healing but not so strong in curing. However, such systems may accommodate both ideas, and this enables them to respond to the introduction of biomedicine in pluralistic contexts while also retaining or needing practices of healing. The distinction therefore is particularly useful when we are looking at issues of change and at problems of "patient satisfaction." The implicit difference between "the physical" and "the psychic" that underlies the distinction needs, however, to be looked at.

3. Body and Mind

A body/mind distinction has been basic to the development of modern philosophy and science in Europe since the time of René Descartes, who elaborated it out of earlier distinctions between body and soul that held sway in medieval times. This is not to argue that Descartes' view simply prevailed either in philosophy or in everyday life. Phenomenological philosophy, for example, stresses greatly what is called the "embodiment" of all thoughts, ideas, experiences, and perceptions that we have; much as everyday life also tells us (see A. J. Strathern 1996). But the distinction itself has proved very important to biomedical science, giving it a powerful materialist cast. Though this has led to enormous scientific advances that still continue through the findings of microbiology, there is at the same time a recognition that health, if seen as a holistic concept, needs to transcend or at least straddle the dichotomy of body and mind, while recognizing that the human organism is an integrated one in which what we label body and mind constantly interact through biochemical mechanisms and that cultural patterns translate into somatic ones and vice-versa. In other words, while we can distinguish between curing and healing, as in 2 above, we need also to realize that curing may depend on emotional states and healing may be influenced by physical states. A holistic approach subsumes both.

Organization of the Book

This book is designed to be read in different ways by academics, general readers with an interest in the cross-cultural study of medicine, and students at either graduate or undergraduate level. For this reason some parts may require a closer acquaintance with medical anthropology than others. In using fairly extended ehtnographic accounts we aim to assist the reader in getting a feel for the topics discussed and to share a baseline of knowledge in terms of which to evaluate the book's heuristic scheme of analysis using the distinctions outlined above. It is not our goal to rival the scope of the textbooks listed in the preceding section in this Introduction. Nevertheless, this book can be used effectively as an introductory and thematic survey in its own terms, and to help academics who use the book for teaching we have supplied at the end of the text lists of questions relating to each chapter. The questions can be either answered from the text or require further thought or reading related to the reader's own knowledge of society.

The book's twelve substantive chapters highlight a number of themes: ideas of the body and humoral systems (Chs. 2 and 3); ritual practices (Chs. 4, 5, and 9); medical pluralism and contemporary circumstances (Ch. 6 and passages in many other chapters, e.g. 2 and 7); and doctor-patient communication in relation to curing and healing (Chs. 8 and 12 as well as other references). In addition, we survey the topics of ethnopsychiatry (Ch. 8), epidemiology (Ch. 10), fertility and reproduction (Ch. 11) and critical medical anthropology (Ch. 13). The conclusions draw together elements from many of these chapters in an analytical scheme illustrating the value of the perspective of curing and healing in medical anthropological studies.

We begin our discussions with ideas of the body, since these are basic to all medical systems and vary cross-culturally. (Some anthropologists argue that "the body" itself is not necessarily a cross-cultural universal. What we are discussing, however, is the body as "embodiment" (Csordas 1994).

Chapter 2

Regimens of Treatment: Humoral Systems (1)

Foster and Anderson, in their classic early survey of medical regimens around the world, developed a basic distinction between personalistic and naturalistic systems of explanation of illness (Foster and Anderson 1978:53–54). In the personalistic system, illness is predominantly traced to actions of malevolent agents such as sorcerers or punitive ones such as ancestors. In the naturalistic system, recourse is had to theories about the properties of the body itself and non-intentional aspects of causation in the cosmos. Both biomedicine and its European precursor, humoral medicine, belong in the latter category, while the beliefs and practices of many of the peoples studied by anthropologists around the world belong to the former. These categorizations are also what we call "ideal types." A given medical system may in practice incorporate elements of both categories, perhaps as a result of historical mixing. Personalistic and humoral ideas can easily be entertained together, whereas biomedical concepts have driven out humoral ones in European mainstream medicine.

Personalistic agents of sickness often stand for moral issues and problems within the community, so that their actions are bound up with the state of people's emotions and these in turn are held to influence the state of their bodies. We therefore have to examine carefully a complex nexus of ideas about the workings of the body, about emotions, about morals, and about spirit and cosmic forces that act in conjunction with emotions and the body to produce sickness, curing, healing, and health. We refer to this whole complex as the "regimen of treatment."

In order to understand how personalistic and humoral ideas can interact, it is useful first to have an idea of what is meant in detail by the category of "humoral" itself. The idea is generally traced to the writings labeled as the Hippocratic corpus, after the Greek physician Hippocrates of Cos, thought to have lived between 460 and 377 B.C. This corpus, in fact, contains lectures and treatises by a number of authors and as Geoffrey Lloyd makes clear in his Introduction to a translation of them, the views of these authors are actually quite discrepant on a number of the issues thought to be diagnostic of the humoral theory (Lloyd 1973: 9). In looking at the corpus overall, it is easy to see how the Hippocratic tradition was an important influence on the development of biomedicine, not via a theory of humors, but because of its pragmatic, empirical, and reasoned approach to problems, based on the importance of direct observation and the recognition of differences among individual patients in terms of their constitutions. Humoral theory was brought into their accounts by some of the Hippocratic writers in order to provide one framework among others in terms of which to organize observation and interpretation as well as the prescription of treatment, but the test they tended to apply to all cures was whether they worked or not. Lloyd further explains this tendency by the fact that doctors at the time were struggling to establish themselves as professionals by attracting fee-paying patients and therefore had to be effective self-promoters, arguing the superiority of their knowledge against that of midwives, herbalists, and charm-sellers, for example. These pragmatic aspects of the Hippocratic tradition survived the decline of humoral ideas and still form an important part of everyday biomedical practice, for instance in the place held by physical examinations of the patient and of bodily excretions.

In spite of this fact, the major legacy of the Hippocratic tradition is generally thought to be the humoral theory of disease and its corresponding treatment by the use of opposites in order to achieve a balancing of the humors. The systematization of this theory owes a good deal to the work of the physician Galen (c. A.D. 129–200), who was a Greek and came from Pergamon in Asia Minor. Galen did his major work in Rome from A.D. 162 onwards, and his work passed into the European world through the writings of Arabic and Persian scholars such as Avicenna and Averroes in the eleventh and twelfth centuries. We need, however, first to go to the Hippocratic writings themselves, specifically to the lecture on physiology called "The Nature of Man," where the author specifies the substances of the human body as blood, phlegm, yellow bile, and black bile. (Commentators have noted that the last is a fictional substance, and that phlegm and yellow bile are signs of pathology whereas blood is not, this perhaps explaining why blood is considered synonymous with health itself in some systems of thought.) Health exists when these substances, the humors, are in correct proportion to each other in terms of their strength and their amount and are well mixed. Good mixing, *eukrasia*, is health, and bad mixing, *dyskrasia*, is sickness, and is also the source of pain. External discharge of a humor causes anxiety, but internal leakage causes greater pain. This theory of the four humors and their balance is opposed to theories that suggest, for example, that blood is the only basic substance.

The author goes on to link this theory to observations regarding the seasons (clearly this extension can apply only when there are seasons). In winter phlegm increases in the body, because both winter and phlegm itself are cold. In spring blood increases and continues to do so in summer, in wet and hot times. During summer and into autumn bile increases, in hot and dry conditions, while blood recedes. Yellow bile predominates in summer, black bile in autumn. A range of diseases are said to spring from the imbalances caused in the humors at different seasons. Excess of one humor has to be met by treatment that will restore the humors to balance, and it follows that physicians must treat disease by the principle of opposition. The mention of the dimensions wet/dry and hot/cold reminds us that the doctrine of the four humors was paralleled by that of the four fundamental elements developed by the philosopher Empedocles of Agrigentum (c. 495–435 B.C.), who declared that there were four "roots," *rhizomata*, earth, water, air, and fire, which create compounds such as blood and bone when they mix in set proportions. (Empedocles also thought that the forces of Love and Strife act on these roots or elements in the cosmos.) The elements in turn were characterized as hot and dry (fire), cold and dry (air), hot and wet (earth) and cold and wet (water). In the Hippocratic corpus this fourfold division into elements is present, but plays its part mostly by way of discussion of the seasons in their interaction with the humors (*chymia*, juices, in Greek).

The complicated intermeshing of quadripartite entities as depicted above is called by anthropologists an *ethnotheory*. Such a theory guides basic ways of thinking when it is transmitted and reproduced culturally. We have to assume that the ideas of the physicians and philosophers we have been outlining were in part systematized by them for their own purposes, but in part also both drew upon and fed into popular thinking and practice at the cultural level. Ethnotheories of this sort do not totally determine what people think, however. In the case of the Hippocratic corpus we have already noted that some writers rejected schematic theorizing and all of them brought in other factors thought to modify the operation of the humors. One such factor was individual variation in the typical mixing of the humors, an idea that later gave rise to a theory of personality types. Another was the medical idea of the importance of diet, exercise, and the control of the inflow and outflow of substances, modulated according to patient characteristics. Here again we find a great emphasis on pragmatism, observation, and experimentation, all aspects which inflect the ethnotheory itself away from any rigid application and into a synergy with experience. These aspects are further tied up with the practical situation of the doctor: he had, as we have seen, to make his ideas and treatments acceptable to his patients. If the theory of humors had been entirely alien to these patients it would not have been usable by the Hippocratic doctors. On the other hand, the theory's application had to be flexible and empirical in order to ensure that it could match up reasonably well with variations in outcome and response.

In terms of practice, then, we find in the corpus considerable stress on the use of diet and exercise to restore health, connected on the one hand with ideas of incorporation/elimination as a means of achieving balance and with the necessity for movement to promote good mixing, *eukrasia*. Such prescriptions are quite closely akin with those stressed today in biomedicine in the sphere of preventive medicine and the promotion of wellness. Again, we may deduce that such treatments made sense to patients because of their own views of the body, as well as influencing in turn those views.

The same must hold for Galen's schemes. Galen was a practical physician who made a living in Rome out of his work. He followed the Hippocratic writings quite closely, as well as admiring Plato, and added to Hippocrates a transcendental view of the beneficence of nature which may be seen as akin to Plato's transcendentalism. Nature was seen as not only orderly by Galen but as craftsmanlike, constructing everything out of the four elements. Disease was seen as unnatural in this sense and health therefore was a state conforming to nature, what in Latin came to be known as the *vis medicatrix naturae*, "the healing power of nature" (Brain 1986: 4). This same state was one of balance, as with the Hippocratic writers. Blood, for example, was held to increase in the spring, as we have seen, but because of spring's temperate qualities this increase was not thought to be harmful. At another season, when blood was thought to be less plentiful, its absence could be harmful, or its intemperate increase could bring sickness, by the theory of *plethora*, overabundance. Kinds and qualities/quantities of food could in turn influence the balance of the humors, especially perhaps the constitution of the blood, a notion we find prevalent even much later, in seventeenth century Italy (Camporesi: 1995: 39), where it was linked to the post-Galenic theory of the four mental temperaments, the sanguine, choleric, phlegmatic, and melancholic (Brain 1986: 7). Since blood was hot and wet, foods having those qualities might be held to increase its quantity in the body.

In the Hippocratic scheme itself, both body and mind were seen as affected by the balance of humors and by the season, so that regimens of food were regarded as important. The treatise on A Regimen for Health suggested diets for all seasons, e.g. that in winter the amount of food eaten should be copious while the fluid intake should be low and consist of undiluted wine. The person should eat bread and roast fish and few vegetables, so as to keep the body warm and dry. Per contra in the summer a person should live on barley cake, quantities of watered wine, and boiled meat, so as to make the body cool and soft in a season that is hot and dry. Balance in the various parts of the body was also seen as important, since the heart, brain, and liver were considered to be dry and hot, wet and cold, and wet and hot: diluted wine in summer would presumably help to keep the heart from becoming too hot and dry.

From practical ethnophysiological and ecological prescriptions of this kind one can understand how a systematics of food could be developed on this basis. The Hippocratic doctors were not engaged in drawing up tables of foods seen as exclusively hot or cold, but in giving advice based on practice, custom, and experience for particular cases. By the time of Celsus (born c. B.C. 25), however, such lists existed, and we find embedded in them elements from Hippocrates, e.g. the idea that boiled meat is cooling and that strong wine is warming (Foster 1994: 7).

We have taken some time to look into the details of the Hippocratic corpus in order to stress its multifaceted, empirically oriented basis, and to use this as a critical prelude to an examination of the idea, discussed by George Foster, in the work just cited, of a "Latin American legacy" derived from Hippocrates. Foster argues that the work of Arab Scholars into which the Hippocratic traditions of medicine were translated was brought by Moslems into Spain and Italy from the end of the seventh century A.D. and became the basis for humoral medicine in Europe in medieval times. Spain, according to Foster, later became the primary source of diffusion of humoral theory to Latin America. We will examine this theme further, but first we give an overview on humoral medicine in Latin America.

Humoral Medicine in
Latin America—An Overview

The term *humoral*, when applied in biotechnical medical systems, refers to a complex immune response utilizing antibodies also known as immunoglobulins. In humoral immunity, these immunoglobulins inactivate, destroy, and/or remove antigens such as viruses. However, in anthropological studies of humoral medical systems, the term refers to a specific and comprehensive organization of concepts about the body and the maintenance of health. In the world today, there are three major variations of humoral theory: traditional Chinese medical practices, Indian Ayurvedic systems, and throughout Latin America humoral beliefs and practices that may differ in their local presentations, but are frequently reduced to concepts in which varying degrees of hot and cold are assigned to foods, activities, emotions, illnesses and therapies. It is important to remember that in the study of these systems, their presentation is often through a synchronic view bounded narrowly in time and space that does not completely convey the subtle variations or the dynamic nature of these practices. The classic Old World models of humoral medicine also utilized assigned qualities of wet/dry, but this is less frequently seen in the Latin American systems. The manner in which medical systems, the physical environment, and their depiction in local metaphors and symbols interrelate may provide clues as to the origin of medical systems (Colson and de Armellada, 1983). The belief that sudden changes in body temperature (immersion in icy water, undue exertion, etc.) can cause illness may be as related to environmental adaptations as it is to specific humoral concepts. As with other long-standing academic debates, it is often left to the interested individual to examine the arguments and evidence presented and arrive at an informed opinion as to their merits and validity.

Throughout the world, health care is pluralistic in nature, that is, people have choices in how, where, and with whom they will seek treatment for health related problems. What constitutes a health problem is often culturally determined, so that in some cultures there is a definite separation between the "mental" and the "physical" (as seen in the Western, Cartesian context) while in others there is a more holistic view of well-being as a balanced state of equilibrium that does not differentiate between the two in terms of either the nature of the problem or the selection of therapeutic interventions. Very often, what has emerged are well-defined, local constructions of patterns in which diseases that have been introduced relatively recently (e.g. with the exposure to new infectious agents and the changes in diet and residence patterns that are introduced with colonization practices) are seen to be best treated by the medical systems that are also newly introduced. Conditions that have been in existence within a society for long periods of time often continue to be treated by indigenous healing systems. These distinctions are rarely as clear-cut as this description seems to indicate. Most often, there is a purposeful and selective blending of options to assure that the best possible outcome will be obtained. With the advent of biotechnical advances in health care, people throughout the world with access to these systems frequently utilize them in the treatment of illnesses. However, in many parts of Latin America, access to hospitals, clinics, and physicians is limited by issues such as geographic isolation and the economics of increasingly privatized health care systems. For many of these people, the hot and cold principles of humoral medicine remain as explanatory models for the causes of illnesses and perhaps, more significantly, as a means of developing practices that have as their goal the maintenance of health. Foster (1994) argues for a less pro-active role in his conclusion that the primary role of humoral theory is "to validate traditional remedies rather than to serve as a guide for treatment" (p. 75).

Humoral systems are characteristically flexible and dynamic. Beliefs and practices vary between individuals, villages, and districts within a country as well as from country to country throughout Latin America. Even within the same settings these concepts may vary across time. The ways in which people organize and integrate their ideas about health and illness and the extent to which differing health-related practices in pluralistic societies are perceived as complementary or antagonistic are often a reflection of culturally mediated ideological beliefs. In a study of illness models subscribed to by some Mestizo populations of the Peruvian Amazon (Kamppinen 1990), three different models were identified: illnesses of God, illnesses due to witchcraft, and illnesses caused by fright. In this system, humoral imbalances are seen as the cause of simple illnesses and while people believe that witchcraft-related illnesses will not respond to biotechnical medicine they may seek biotechnical resolution for the simple illnesses. When simultaneous treatment is sought from ideologically different sources, conflicts can arise when there are contradictions between therapeutic recommendations that will require modification of both or rejection of one or the other. People usually base their choices on what they believe will be the most efficacious treatment, but these beliefs are based in larger cultural belief systems and frequently influenced by socioeconomic constraints. In cultures in which there are high degrees of social stratification, the relationships between different medical systems often reflect larger, societal patterns of inequalities (Pedersen and Baruffati 1989). The ideologies surrounding choice in health issues can also be viewed within the context of the process of socialization and as such may be utilized as a means of expressing resistence to domination. In this view, the concept of "mutuality" as described by James Scott will assume importance within a subordinated group. Thus, shared indigenous beliefs surrounding the causes and treatment of illnesses will be "practiced, articulated, enacted, and disseminated" within social spaces that have been created and are defined as autonomous from the dominant spaces (Scott 1990).

In her examination of medical pluralism in Bolivia, Crandon-Malamud notes the merging of indigenous Aymara beliefs with the causative and humoral concepts associated with Hispanic folk medicine. For example, the causes of illness may, at times, be attributed to magic. The Aymara of the altiplano may attribute illness and misfortune to the failure to appease (with offerings of meat, alcohol, and other gifts) the phantom known as the *khan achachi* (Crandon-Malamud 1991). At other times, people will utilize knowledge and beliefs that originated in Hispanic traditions. This merging of Aymara and Hispanic traditions will additionally be incorporated with biomedical etiological and therapeutic concepts. People may have a view of distinct, separate systems of evaluation and treatment and of the manner in which they navigate through these systems, but when and how they choose one system over the others (or elements from each one) will be determined by well-defined belief systems, socioeconomic realities, and temporal constraints. In some places, including the Bolivian altiplano, there may or may not be a clear distinction between biomedicine and indigenous practices, and the latter are also syncretic blends of different, local systems. In humoral systems, there is an assignment of hot or cold characteristics in a way that establishes oppositional values that can then be utilized to address states of perceived disequilibrium. In his discussion of humoral medicine in Guatemala, Michael H. Logan (1973) noted that the designation of something as hot or cold is not a reflection of any intrinsic physical quality of an object or action but more to "the constitutional essence or innate character of a given item or personal state of being" (p. 387). For example, 79% of the respondents in a survey conducted in Tzintzuntzan, Mexico classified ice as hot (Foster 1994). And in Guatemala, diseases such as meningitis and pneumonia (which are frequently associated with high fevers) are classified as cold (Logan 1973). One of the ways in which these characteristics are assigned is described by Frank Lipp (1991) in his study of the Mixe of Oaxaca in southwestern Mexico:

> Medicinal plants are classified as being hot, cold, and neutral. Any plant sharp to the taste, such as pine, is considered to be "hot," and "hot" plants with a burning sensation are considered to be poisonous. Plants with a bitter taste are "neutral." In the second test, if the leaf feels hot on the forehead, the plant is "cold." If nothing is felt, it is "hot" or "neutral." "Cold" plants are used to treat sicknesses such as rheumatism; "hot" plants are used for fever and chills (p.186).

In all humoral-based systems, there is the recognition that excesses in either quality are disruptive to a desired state of homeostasis or balance and that to maintain or restore balance it is necessary to manipulate one's exposure to hot and cold influences. This is not to say that simple illness/treatment dichotomies exist, that, for example, if one has experienced an excess of hot it can always be balanced by the application of cold. People who are perceived to be in a state of disequilibrium that has been defined as hot (for example, excessive anger, pregnancy, heavy work) may also be seen as especially vulnerable to illness if exposed to activities, things, or states of being that are categorized as cold (bathing, certain foods and medicines), but in general, excessive states of either hot or cold or the over-indulgence in foods designated as one or the other creates a state of extreme susceptibility to illness and disequilibrium which can be mediated by the judicious application of things that are perceived not to be threatening (i.e. excessively hot *or* cold). At times, temporarily refraining from any activity or the ingestion of all food or drink is the manner in which excesses may by moderated.

In some systems, there are illnesses that can be caused by both hot or cold insults. For example, Foster (1994) describes the etiology of diarrhea as either the result of a "flooding" of hot bile from the gall bladder into the stomach following an emotional shock or because of an over-ingestion of "cold" food such as broad bean soup or ice cream. In Lima, Peru, diarrhea is seen as an "invasion" of the body by cold or as the result of the ingestion of "cold" foods (Escobar, Salazar, and Chuy 1983). The implications of these beliefs may be significant. The rejection of an infectious explanatory model for some cases of diarrhea may result in practices that will promote its spread or result in treatments that may affect the outcome in an adverse way, for example in the avoidance of foods that contain essential nutrients in cases of infantile diarrhea.

Pregnancy is almost universally classified as a "hot" state. In the historical view of the Aztecs, this was demonstrated by a prohibition against a pregnant woman serving a drink known as *pulque* (classified as cold) because it was believed she would rob it of its intoxicating qualities (Ortiz de Montellano 1990). The humoral perception of pregnancy as a hot state is, in some part, attributed to the concept of an increase in the amount of blood in a pregnant woman's body (in biotechnical medicine there are related principles in which hormonal and thermodynamic changes result in, among other things, increased circulating volume in the cardiovascular systems of pregnant women). Because of her hot state, a pregnant woman will be protected against things that are considered to be excessively cold such as beans, pork, and sodas. Midwives practicing in Guatemala will utilize herbal teas that have been assigned hot or cold properties as well as therapeutics such as massage to restore humoral equilibrium in a pregnant woman. These treatments are especially utilized in the event of a "stress" such as the experience of excessive anger or fright (Cosminsky and Scrimshaw 1980). Throughout Latin America, many of the behaviors that are beneficial to the health of pregnant women and the developing fetus have at their foundation concepts that are governed by humoral systems.

As with all medical systems, human beliefs and the culture surrounding diseases and illness may cause people to make modifications that are less than advantageous. In biotechnical medicine an example of this is the manner in which people interpret ideas about vitamin therapies. Despite extensive research in this area, it is difficult to find consensus between physicians about the use of these supplements, and taken to an extreme, excessive fat-soluble vitamins are dangerous and can induce serious illnesses. Humoral medicine and its tenets have existed for long periods of time and are, for the most part, principles that directly contribute to the maintenance of equilibrium and, in the case of illness, to the restoration of health.

Foster's Theory: Personalistic and Naturalistic Thinking

We have argued that humoral medicine is naturalistic in its focus but can also accommodate personalistic elements. It is exactly such an accommodation that we find in Latin America. For example, witchcraft or the evil eye can be thought of as working through the disruption of balance in bodily humors. The two classes of influence are thus brought together in terms of an idea of different causes working together rather than being separated as exclusive and competing theories of illness. But where this happens we cannot truly say that medical thought and practice is Hippocratic, because to do so would be to belie the elements of empirical scientific investigation enshrined in the Hippocratic outlook. At the same time, the Latin American case might correspond to the state of popular thinking in Greece in the fifth and fourth centuries B.C. The Hippocratic corpus provides for a particular kind of regimen of treatment, based on naturalistic modes of thinking, in which all the emphasis is on manipulating the body's constituents and condition. Personalistic thinking, however, tends to stress counteraction against the agents who have caused or sent the disease. It implies in principle a different regimen of diagnosis and treatment. When the two ways of thinking are combined we may expect some complicated results. We may also expect, however, that a complex scheme such as we find in Hippocrates will be selectively rather than totally appropriated.

It is this process of selective appropriation that attracted Foster's interest. He argues, first, that the introduction of humoral ideas into the New World came about through the work of the Spanish elite—physicians and clergymen—whose ideas then filtered down to the masses. The modes of transmission included hospitals, the missionary orders, pharmacies, and home medical guides (*recetarios*) that were made widely available in the colonial period (Foster 1994: 155). Second, he notes that the humoral system, as adopted, tended to preserve the hot/cold dichotomy and either to drop the wet/dry dimension or assimilate it into the hot/cold scheme, a process he attributes to the difficulties of preserving the whole scheme in a context of illiteracy. Regardless of this last point, which is debatable, it does seem that the hot/cold dimension was the most appealing or encompassing, and it seems quite possible that it meshed easily enough with indigenous concepts in cases (such as the Aztec) where an opposition of this kind also existed culturally. Further, the Spanish colonizers brought with them both prestige and power and the colonized may have accepted humoral ideas of medicine as they did Catholic ideas of theology, grafting these where possible onto their own ethnotheories of life and death. We might even suggest that the colonizers sought to find in indigenous cultures points of similarity with their own, on which they may have seen themselves as building in order to create "higher" forms, a process that can go hand in hand with also setting out putative cultural differences. For humoral theory to be adopted, however, the schema of the humors themselves needs to have been transmitted in conjunction with hot/cold classifications and the treatment of disease by opposites. From Foster's own extended work in Tzintzuntzan, Mexico, it appears that the hot/cold dimension (whether seen as thermal or as metaphorical) is what predominates in ideas about the body, not the idea of the four humors themselves. So it is a stripped-down humoral theory indeed if it is not based on the Hippocratic idea of the humors as such. Of course other substances may be thought to be in play, and ideas about blood, at any rate, are important (as they are also in many other cultures where a strictly humoral theory of the body is not at work). The overall effect of a stress on the hot/cold dimension is to privilege the arena of food qualities as a predominant means of treating forms of sickness, along with attempts to alter the ambient environment of the sick person by keeping it warm or cool. (This last point also raises the question of whether "a humoral system" depends on the metaphorical attribution of heat, as Foster argues, over and above thermal attributions. We may suggest that the thermal leads into the metaphorical, and also that a great deal of pragmatism enters precisely here, since if an illness is seen as cold the foods customarily prescribed to be given to patients suffering from it will themselves be classified as hot.)

That there is a conventional aspect to attributions is clear when we consider that emotions are also described in hot/cold terms in Tzintzuntzan. Anger, fright, and envy are thought to make the body hot by an upsurge of bile into the blood. In the case of envy, the person experiencing the emotion does not become sick but rather endangers the object of the envy by casting the evil eye, *mal de ojo*, a form of witchcraft. We reach the point here of seeing how in a specific case a personalistic and naturalistic theory have intersected, in this case via ideas of the emotions. These in turn imply moral and ethical judgements, so we move into the domain of intersection between illness and morality, as occurs readily in personalistic systems of thought.

We will see exemplifications of this point when we look next at some ways in which humoral ideas, as broadly defined, operate in some Latin American contexts. It is true that humoral thinking feeds easily into biomedicine in one respect, since it imputes naturalistic causes to sickness and prescribes, or validates, material treatments such as herbs as well as particular kinds of food. Foster comments (1994: 77): "there is little or no concern with social dimensions of causality. The individual's concern is to stay healthy, not to keep his social relationships in good order." However, he does note that in the case of witchcraft "who" and "why" questions are asked; and in his earlier textbook written with Barbara Anderson he gives case-materials from Mexican contexts that show the condition of *susto*, soul-loss by fright, in close implication with social and moral issues between people. In one case a Mexican-American couple with six children of their own suffered from overcrowding caused by a prolonged visit of the husband's relatives. The wife began to suffer from shortness of breath and sweating; her sister and two godmothers diagnosed *susto*, later confirmed by a local *curandera* (female curer). The relatives were then asked to leave and shortly thereafter she recovered. In another case a young woman scolded her drunk husband, who beat her and put her out into the rain. She walked to her mother's house, and was taken to a *curandera*, since it was feared that her child, through the prenatal experience of the beating, would after its birth suffer from *susto* (Foster and Anderson 1979: 149, 152).

No mention is made of humoral correlates of *susto* here, and Foster regards notions of soul-loss as outside of the humoral system as such, but the point is that these notions are entertained by the same people who also use humoral ideas, so that it is quite possible they think of *susto* as an example of the general "loss of balance" within the body, through the temporary departure of the soul. It is more plausible to suppose that there are bridging elements between humoral (naturalistic) and non-humoral (personalistic) systems of belief when these co-occur among the same people than it is to suppose that no connections are made. Nevertheless, it is true that such connections, if present, appear to be muted in ethnographic accounts. Personalistic elements can be seen as predominantly Pre-Hispanic, so it may be that their relative paucity of articulation with naturalistic ones reflects the limits of blending or syncretism as against contextually defined co-existence. Connections are, however, present in certain domains. Janis Jenkins and Martha Valiente, writing of El Salvador, report on women's experience of *calor* (heat) in terms of surges of *corrientes* (electric currents), *fuego* (fire) or *llama* (flame), as a result of fear and worry or anger, among other things. *Calor* is thus an embodiment of emotion which can also accompany *susto* (fright, soul-loss), and *susto* is a condition strongly influenced by social relations. One woman suffered from it as a result of the disapproving and unresponsive looks of her husband (Jenkins and Valiente 1994: 168–172). Authors usually see *susto* as pre-Hispanic and *calor* as a Hispanic idea, so here we see their clear contemporary influence. Hugo Nutini and Jack Roberts, in their magisterial study of blood-sucking witchcraft in rural Tlaxcala, Mexico, also note that the activities of sorcerer-curers known as *tetlachihuic* were largely based on a form of sympathetic-homeopathic-contagious magic which we can see as separate from humoral notions. But they were thought to have the ability to effect many bodily changes through the use of *tlapaltizolitzi* powers consisting of strong "airs" which they could also use to counteract the sleep-inducing "vapor" wielded by witches. Nutini and Roberts further observe that "the widespread distinction in Mesoamerica between hot (*caliente*) and cold (*frío*) foods is extended in rural Tlaxcala to bodily and psychological states. In this context the *tetlachihuic*'s craft is mainly concerned with the confrontation and contraposition of hot and cold states (Nutini and Roberts

1993: 52, 66)." Thus, sorcerers at any rate are portrayed as operating at least partly in terms of the same dimensions of hot and cold that predominate in the humoral system of medicine and they also act as curers as well as killers.

Furst, in her discussion of the soul, *fonalli*, in Ancient Mexico, propounds the idea that the soul must be kept warm otherwise the person will die, and notes that soul loss was thought to disturb the hot/cold balance in the body (Furst 1995: 31). Correcting over-psychologized accounts of *susto*, she cites the theory that it may represent hypoglycemia (low blood sugar), chronic illness, and poor diet (p. 122), and suggests that the preoccupation with temperature balance and health seen in the hot/cold classifications of the New World need not have been derived from European humoral medicine but may be indigenous, although blending between the indigenous and introduced notions undoubtedly occurred. Against the stress on the metaphorical by Foster she anchors her argument in physiology, the environment, epidemiology, and evidence from the past. If this viewpoint has merit, it turns Foster's view upside down. It is not that humoral thinking brought an arbitrary set of hot/cold distinctions to the Americas. It is rather that these were already in place there and indeed were perhaps more systematized than in the Hippocratic corpus and they therefore structured the absorption of Hispanic notions by rejecting the wet/dry dimension in favor of the fundamental hot/cold idea representing the difference between life and death (p. 124). The question of "intersection" between humoral and non-humoral ideas would in this perspective disappear, since the non-humoral ideas of the soul turn out to be both humoral in a sense and also, however, pre-Hispanic.

Similar considerations appear when we move into other regimens of treatment that show affinities with the Hippocratic system in terms of notions of balance in the body, as we shall see if we turn to work done in Japan.

Japan: Holism, Pluralism, and *Kanpo* Medicine

Margaret Lock (1980) has studied medical pluralism in Japan. Her perspectives on biomedicine derive from her work on the holistic traditions of Southeast Asian medicinal systems. Her most detailed work has been carried out in urban contexts in Japan, where she has shown the interplay between the introduced practice of biomedicine and the Chinese system of *Kanpo* or herbal medicine. Lock points to a relatively equal cooperation between the two systems with easy referral from one to the other. This is made more effective by the rule that *Kanpo* practitioners should be trained in biomedicine, hence they are doctors who understand both systems. *Kanpo* has therefore fared much better in Japan than has "folk" medicine in western Europe since the bias in favor of biomedical practices developed. Several factors are involved: *Kanpo* has come to stand for "Japanese culture"; it is recognized for insurance purposes; and it is an agreeable therapy for older patients with long-term chronic conditions who can make frequent, almost social visits to herbal clinics; and above all the herbal regimen suits Japanese ideas of the body and its needs. Biomedical treatment is seen as invasive and aggressive, especially in the form of surgery, whereas herbal medicines are seen more as foods, nourishing the body and helping to restore the balance of substances within it.

Lock traces the historical movements of medicinal ideas in Japan. Japanese contact with Chinese ideas was primarily via Korea, whence in the fourth century A.D. Chinese books were imported into the country by scholars. Korean doctors then set up treatment practices within Japan. After 601 A.D., Buddhism was declared acceptable in China and spread to Japan. The Japanese Ministry of Health set up in 702 A.D. had a section "The Bureau of Yin Yang," and through this Confucian philosophical ideas were introduced into the country. Chinese herbal medicines were also accepted, but obtaining the raw materials to fill the prescriptions was often difficult. During this time, Buddhist, Confucian, and Taoist ideas about the body and wellness mingled together and fire, water, air, and earth were accepted as the elements of matter. Buddhism was later suppressed from 1569 onwards and Confucianism stressed. Many different schools of medical thought were arising , e.g. of *goseiha* (mild) and *kohoha* (strong) medicine. Unlicensed doctors continued to practice a mixture of *Kanpo* and folk medicine. *Kanpo* is the term that refers to the entire medical system brought to Japan from China in the sixth century. The word means "Chinese method." In modern Japan it is also used to refer to herbal medicine but not to acupuncture, moxibustion (a technique in which small cones of a powdered plant, mugwort, are burned on the body at particular points thought to have heightened therapeutic significance), or massage (pp. 15, 50–66).

Cosmopolitan medicine began to gain ground in the 19th century with a decision in 1824 to introduce smallpox vaccination and in 1869 to adopt the German system of medical education. In 1876 the government ruled that all doctors must study western medicine but there were 23,000 *Kanpo* doctors and only about 520 registered cosmopolitan doctors in 1873. At this time competitive pressure on *Kanpo* medicine increased and it became a folk and home remedy practice with avoidance of doctors being the primary aim, except against smallpox, tuberculosis, and for wounds. The competitive context made for secrecy between different professional schools, and there was much pragmatic innovation. In 1914 the Kitasato Research Institute was built in Japan to carry out research on medicine, and in 1974 a branch devoted to East Asian medicine was set up. In 1976 a law was passed allowing the use of herbal prescriptions again (pp. 61–66).

Lock notes the swing of the pendulum back towards holism in medicine that went along with a recognition of ecological factors in industrial societies like Japan, in addition to a greater understanding that therapy has to rely on cultural symbols in order to be effective. She distinguishes between Cosmopolitan, East Asian, Folk, and Popular medical systems in Japan. Cosmopolitan Medicine is what we would classify as Western biomedicine. East Asian Medicine includes *Kanpo*, acupuncture, moxibustion, and massage. Folk medicine includes treatment at Shinto shrines and Buddhist temples. Popular Medicine includes self-medication in the home. In general, health standards in Japan are high and there is an aging population which heavily utilizes these health care facilities. Doctors get reimbursement on a points system for seeing patients, and this gives an incentive to allow return visits of patients which the elderly seem to take advantage of (pp. 1–20).

Buddhist priests who first brought *Kanpo* medicine to Japan took over from Shinto priests who interceded with gods and were concerned with issues of purity and pollution. Prior to 200 B.C. actual practitioners of medicine were shamans. After this, Confucian influences came into play, with the idea of secular balance and maintenance of good relations with one's family. Concepts of yin/yang were employed, yin being feminine and contractive, yang being masculine and expansive. Equilibrium was considered to be the ideal for well-being. Disease was thought to arise when the body became out of balance. Also, there was thought to exist an exchange of energy, *ch'i* or *ki*, between the body and the environment and within the body. This energy was thought to flow in prescribed routes. At certain seasons a noxious substance could enter the body while one's resistance was low, remain dormant, and manifest itself at a later season (p. 37). Diagnosis was and is still done with the aid of palpation in which pulses are read at different points along the wrists. These pulses signify the state of different organs within the body at large. Treatment of disease is thus intended to restore balance and harmony within the body and between the body and the environment. Treatment may use the *gosei* system which is based on the cold/hot (= yin/yang) distinction and treatment is by opposites. Thus, conditions that are categorized as hot (yang state) are treated with medicines that are categorized as cold. Likewise conditions that are considered to be caused by the yin state are treated with medicines that are thought to be hot. Another system of treatment is the *gomi* system which employs a classification of five tastes (acid, bitter, sweet, pungent, or salty) thought to affect five relevant groups of body organs.

There are many different combinations of medicines, individually tailored to treat various conditions. Also, acupuncture and moxibustion are used on pressure points in the body, as well as massage to restore balance. In East Asian Medicine, therapy is mild and allows the body itself to do the hard work of reestablishing balance and thus healing (pp. 27–49).

Non-verbal techniques of nurturance are used in socializing children. The mother's control is expected to be gentle but persistent manipulation. Verbal explanations are not considered necessary. Babies are kept quiet, rather than stimulated, but frequent contact with a human body is maintained and children often sleep with their parents past weaning. The mother is more closely identified with the child than the father. As children grow up they are expected to behave in a neat, clean, and calm fashion. At some time they can *amaeru*, presume on the love of others, though not verbally. Sickness is one way to get that love and to be free of responsibilities for a while. Dependency on the mother continues in adulthood. A young wife takes her new child back to her own mother for guidance. Sick leave from work is generous and seniors indulge juniors regarding sickness.

People talked readily to Lock about sickness and the condition of their bodies. The concept of *ki*, human emotions in a situation of continuous flux, is very important. Illnesses "from" *ki* produce bodily symptoms; "of" *ki* mental ones; the expression "*ki* has changed" refers to psychotic symptoms. People are socialized to manage their *ki*. *Hara*, stomach, is also important, and there is a corresponding concern with stomach cancer. There is a large number of stomach medicines. The center of gravity or *tanden* of the body is thought to be in the region of the navel. *Hara* also has a mental significance, functioning as "mind" or "heart" do in English. Tension is manifested first in the stomach and wearing of stomach bands to "hold oneself together" is common. In general, the Shinto religious background shows very strongly in continuing attitudes towards pollution. Gauze masks and sweat baths as forms of protection and purification have both to be seen in this light. There are also rules for foods which should not be eaten together (e.g. mushrooms and spinach). A survey of families showed that visits to religious practitioners are made by both upper and lower middle classes, especially for birth rituals (Shinto), but not as an alternative to going to a doctor. Acupuncture and moxibustion are used as well as *Kanpo* and cosmopolitan medicine. In some cases people will consult fortune-tellers as well as doctors, especially if illness is severe and prognosis uncertain. Shinto shrines may be visited or people attend one of the new religions which have proliferated in Japan during the Post World War II period (pp. 83–107).

At the *Kanpo* clinic patients may have to wait to see a doctor, but the waiting room is pleasant and when they do see the doctor they receive personal attention. The detection of points of imbalance of the body in relation to the total environment is important; pulses are taken in East Asian style. Advice is given regarding diet and lifestyle, which is good for ulcers. Psychosomatic elements in conditions are recognized. There is a high incidence of chronic conditions in those treated. The comments of patients are revealing: "These doctors look at me carefully and they listen to what I have to say. I like the combination of science and herbs. Here they treat me like a whole person and not like a machine." Informants — especially those over forty — also thought that "not keeping the rules of life correctly" produced illness (pp. 111–126).

Kanpo doctors do not reject biomedical theories but they believe in the Taoist idea of keeping the body in balance with the environment. Their approach is ecological and homeostatic. They see people as either yin (passive) or yang (active) types. They are sensitive to effects of climate on disease (as were the Hippocratic doctors in ancient Greece). Biomedical diagnosis is accepted at the cellular level, and the East Asian approach at the level of the whole body or person. Cosmopolitan diagnosis is used to define diseases that cannot be treated by *Kanpo* (pp. 127–143).

The herbal medicines themselves largely come from China, and their use is becoming more expensive as the Chinese raise prices. Doses vary with the patient's own strength and weakness and with their yin/yang state. In some cases patients are encouraged to help mix their own medicine as a part of the medicinal process. No factor is considered primarily responsible for illness. "Correlative thinking" holds, that is doctors look for whole complexes of symptoms and try to see how these are related to the total state of the body in the cosmos. Doctors do not attempt to change conditions of stress in patient's lives but help them to adjust to it biochemically. Patients are never told there is nothing wrong with them. The doctors themselves have chosen to work at the clinic as a result of cures they or their family experienced. They also think that the patient can be his/her own doctor and that there is an intuitively creative element in medicine. They tend to practice Japanese arts such as judo and to insist on eating natural Japanese food to stay healthy themselves and to be able to treat others (pp. 144–154).

Japan: Culture, "Japanese Germs," and the Body

It is interesting to compare Margaret Lock's materials with those of another medical anthropologist, Emiko Ohnuki-Tierney, who uses the perspectives of both an insider, since by birth she is Japanese, and an outsider, since she has been trained and teaches in her adopted society, the

United States of America. Ohnuki-Tierney stresses both the influence of culture generally in constructions of illness and the specifics of Japanese ideas about the body.

Ohnuki-Tierney records that she had been living in America since 1958, when she was in her early teens, and had carried out fieldwork among the Ainu people of Hokkaido prior to 1979 when she first decided to go back to her own area, Kobe, to study patterns of health care there. She notes that on her first re-entry, the Kobe people "seemed strange, with intriguing behavioral patterns and thought processes," but after a while she became reaccustomed and decided to return to America before carrying out a second phase of fieldwork in 1980, aiming to reach a balanced perspective (Ohnuki-Tierney 1984: 16). She does indeed achieve this goal, combining the use of categories salient for the Kobe people themselves with her own further reflections on these based on anthropological theory.

One of these categories deals with the concept of space specifically in relation to hygiene. In particular, she notes that the Japanese express an extremely overt concern with a distinction between the "outside" and the "inside," as applied especially to the house. The house inside must be kept pure and clean, while the outside is seen as polluting and dirty. People who enter a house wash their hands to remove the dirt from outside, including the "dirt" of other people (*hitogomi*). As she notes, people explain this in terms of a modern theory of germs, but there are germs inside houses too. She cites the theoretician Claude Lévi-Strauss here, who pointed out that an "indigenous model" may act as a screen to conceal a deeper reality. The idea of germs conceals the deeper notions of purity and pollution applied to space. Hence she arrives at her concept of "Japanese germs" (1984: 17, 21–50). We may comment further that the germ model is recent in Japanese culture, a result of biomedical influence, while the purity/pollution concepts belong to the ancient Shinto stratum of Japanese culture. Prior to the introduction of biomedicine there would have been no need to overlay the earlier indigenous model with another one that concealed it. The need to do so arose from the ascendancy of biomedicine as a paradigm, an ascendancy that has itself more recently been tempered by the revived popularity of *Kanpo*, Chinese herbal medicine, as discussed by Lock.

One of the illustrations in Ohnuki-Tierney's book (1984: 23) shows the *genkan*, the entrance lobby to a middle-class Japanese house where outside footgear must be removed and left and inside footwear put on. This is indeed a very rigid rule. Breaking it will provoke cries of consternation and remonstrance against the ignorant (and surely foreign) guest who commits such an error. Children are carefully socialized into these rules. On buses and trains they must take off their shoes if they want to sit on the seats. On commuter trains if one places a briefcase on the floor, it will be lifted up and placed instead in an overhead compartment. Taxi drivers wear gloves, and people readily wear masks. All these actions reveal a sensitivity to dirt that belongs especially to outside contexts, and efforts not to communicate such dirt between human bodies. Cars may be taken to a shrine on New Year's Day to have them purified. (There are similar customs in Scotland about washing off the dirt of the Old Year on New Year's Eve.) The inside area of a habitation may extend to its yard wall: the inner part of the wall is kept pure, but the householder is not concerned about the wall's outer surface. Gateways are meeting places of the outside and the inside, and people returning from a funeral must purify themselves with a sprinkling of salt at the yard gateway before re-entering their home (Ohnuki-Tierney 1984: 25).

Sensitivity to dirt extends to practices in regard to eating. Using the hands for eating is suspect and chopsticks, defined as clean, are used. Japanese people may find it uncomfortable in particular to eat sandwiches with their hands just after they have used money, which is defined as particularly unclean since it passes through human hands constantly (p. 29). Chopsticks are reversed if used to take food from a common dish so as not to contaminate the dish with saliva. (This example shows that the "inside" fluids of the body can also be seen as unclean.)

Another category used by Ohnuki-Tierney is physiomorphism, a term she uses instead of somatization. Physiomorphism also refers to an aspect of behavior and experience that is widely, if not uniformly, signaled in contemporary anthropology by the term *embodiment*. Both physiomorphism and embodiment refer to broad ideas about the body, including its health. In accorance with this notion Ohnuki-Tierney stresses that the term *ki* (glossed as mind, spirit, energy, and discussed also by Lock and many others) does not refer to a domain of psychology, as it might be understood in Western terms. Putting this another way, we may argue it does not refer to a mind/body opposition or separation. Rather it refers, as she notes, to an "imbalance created in the body" (p. 75). Chill winds, inborn constitutions seen in terms of nerves and "blood types," and agents such as aborted fetuses may all be involved in causing such an imbalance. Apparently, this concern with balance does not extend to issues of the emotions. This is striking, given the prevalence of such notions in etiologies around the world. Some anthropologists have suggested that where overt reference to emotional upsets is not a cultural practice, these are covertly shown in bodily symptoms, i.e. in somatization. Ohnuki-Tierney, however, objects to the implications of this term, from her dual outsider/insider perspective. First, as an insider she wants to present the Japanese views themselves, not translate them into terms appropriate to a different world view. Second, she argues that it is not only the body that is in focus, since other material agents may be seen as at work in producing effects on the body. We return to this conflict of opinion below, noting only that in relation to Japanese germs she does look beneath the indigenous categories for a deeper reality but here declines to do so. Nevertheless, the ethnographic point she makes is well taken.

Japanese physiomorphism, in her usage, would correspond to a naturalistic version of humoral theory. For example, nerves (*shinkei*) are cited as agents of sickness, but these are nerves in a physiological, not a psychological sense, and are treated with bathing, massage, and acupuncture as attempts to restore balance to the body. Blood type is also cited as a cause of illness, and here the term refers to inborn constitutions and personality types, not strictly to serological types as recognized in biomedicine. Blood type seems to function as humoral type. Constitutions can also be classified as acid or alkaline, correlating further with categories of foods (e.g. meat is acid, vegetables are alkaline), and it is thought that the human body is at its best when it is slightly alkaline. Too much meat makes it overacidic, and the levels are described in popular literature in terms of pH values. This, like many other touches, shows how humoral ideas have been modernized or legitimized by the addition of biomedical or scientific notions, given a novel twist. Acidic constitutions are said to lead to diseases like cancer or ulcers. Sesame is seen as an important health food because it is alkaloid and thus counteracts acidity. The idea of balance is therefore central here again, showing a clear correspondence with Hippocratean concepts.

Ohnuki-Tierney classifies another etiological agent in with physiomorphism: the aborted fetus. Such fetuses are given a memorial service, and tombs for them can be purchased if these can be afforded. If not, the parents may buy a posthumous name for the fetus and this is written on a tablet which is included in the family's ancestral alcove to which offerings are made. The fetus thus acquires a kind of posthumous personhood. Prayers and apologies are made in written form to such fetuses, mostly signed by the mother. There is an idea that these fetuses, being innocent of sin, are easily reborn. Such an idea might help to relieve the sense of guilt that appears to underlie the practice of apologizing to the fetuses and the incidence of what Ohnuki-Tierney identifies as mild psychosomatic illness experienced by their mothers. Here, then, she is saying that the fetus stands instead of the feeling of guilt as the recognized agent of the mother's feeling illness, and that this exemplifies again physiomorphism and an aversion to psychotherapy. Still, the idea of guilt does seem to be consciously recognized in the practice of apologizing. The fetus is also not exactly blamed for the mother's illness. Ohnuki-Tierney stresses (p. 86) that physiomorphism eliminates "the possibility of blaming another person for misfortune" while privileging the basic idea that health = balance and sickness = imbalance. If she is right in her assessment, it is clear that even though the aborted fetus ideas resemble notions of personalistic causation of sickness, they operate very differently from those in which personalistic agents act in association with the moral order and with the emotions of people as they are perceived by the actors themselves, such as we find in Mount Hagen and other places in New Guinea (see Ch. 3). It is also clear that Ohnuki-Tierney feels as an observer that the idea of physiomorphism does operate sometimes to obscure what we might call the psychic correlates of illness. It therefore acts as Arthur Kleinman argued somatization does in the case of the Chinese, i.e. as the manifestation of emotional distress and disorder through physical symptoms that can then be treated physically by medicines (see Kleinman 1980 and further discussion of this theme in our Ch. 8 on Ethnopsychiatry in this book). If this is correct, it helps also to explain the great popularity of *Kanpo* herbal medicine, since it answers to the humoral basis of Japanese physiomorphism more exactly than does western biomedicine.

Ohnuki-Tierney devotes a chapter to *Kanpo* (1984: 91–122). She stresses the significance of the concept of *shōkōgun*, clusters of symptoms and prodromes that may produce illness but do not necessarily correspond to any single disease. The *Kanpo* doctor examines the patient's body closely and asks about habits, relying heavily on visual, olfactory, and tactile evidence. Anything seen as showing an imbalance adds to the *shōkōgun*, along with the patient's own statements and with the physician's perception of the patient's overall constitution and the environment in which the patient lives. The *shōkōgun* thus shows the sum of factors relating to imbalance and medicines are prescribed and mixed to restore balance in complex ways. Disease pathogenesis is not in focus, hence drugs are not used to target specific conditions. For example, a fibroma is not seen as an illness but as a result of unbalanced blood circulation, which must therefore be corrected. The medicines prescribed to restore balance must themselves be mixed and balanced carefully so as to fit the whole *shōkōgun* and not to upset the patient's body. Ohnuki-Tierney observes (p. 99) that *Kanpo* has been most successful in treating chronic and degenerative conditions such as diabetes, but has also been used for arthritis, neuralgia, shoulder stiffness, and chilling (the last seen as a condition of blood). It works well also in many contexts where its presuppositions are shared by doctors and patients alike. Ohnuki-Tierney observes that this gives *Kanpo* a certain strength in Japan by contrast with biomedicine, and here she quotes the concept that is central to our own discussions in this book, the distinction made by Fabrega and others between disease and illness. "In any contemporary society there is a culture of medical professionals who diagnose and treat *disease*, and a culture of people who experience *illness*" (p. 101). If so, biomedicine has gradually increased the gap between professionals and patients, whereas in *Kanpo* medical practice the gap is minimized. Does this mean, then, that *Kanpo* heals or attempts to heal while biomedicine seeks to cure?

Curing and Healing: Some Reflections

Curing refers to the treatment of specific conditions, seen as diseases; healing to restoring wellness to the body or person as a whole. Margaret Lock's discussion of East Asian medicine, including *Kanpo*, suggests that such medicine is based on holistic ideas of wellness, premised on the restoration of balance in the body and the avoidance of aggressive interventions that may themselves upset such a balance. From this viewpoint, *Kanpo* is about healing. Ohnuki-Tierney's discussion of the idea of the *shōkōgun*-symptom cluster and its treatment by mixtures of herbs supports this interpretation also. On the other hand, holism tends to mean to the western reader the unity of mind, body, and spirit. Ohnuki-Tierney's argument here is that Japanese physiomorphism excludes an explicit consideration of the mind seen as psyche, or of the emotions as involved in producing sickness. From this aspect, then, we might conclude that *Kanpo* is about curing, not healing in the broader sense, even though the specific ideas about illness conditions do not correspond exactly with western concepts of disease. The Japanese case therefore shows that complex aspects of both curing and healing may be combined within a single broad cultural context, and that categorizations in terms of either of these two ideas are themselves dependent on the aspects under review and one's interpretation of them.

India: Ayurvedic Medicine

The materials on Japan have shown us overlaps with, but also differences from, the Hippocratic regimen of medicine. We continue this comparison by looking at data from India. Ayurvedic medicine — knowledge (*veda*) for prolonging (*ayus*), the continuation of life — has several distinct traditions: (1) An elaborate and comprehensive system of classification of bodily and environmental phenomena that considers that no illness occurs randomly but as a result of a particular infraction of set rules of order expounded in ancient texts. (2) A reliance on the subjective experience of the body and Ayurveda texts which refer to organs, substances, and structures that do not correspond to actual human anatomy. (3) A common classificatory pattern that relies on two kinds of land types: one being wet, dark, and low and the other being dry, light, and high (Trawick 1995: 282–284).

Ayurvedic texts can be divided into two types of works: *samhita*, treatises on medicine, and *nighantu*, dictionaries of *materia medica*. These two belong to different literary genres and different periods, the *nighantu* appearing later. In Ayurvedic thought this has been considered to derive from the beliefs about the consumption of food raised on these two types of land, called in Sanskrit *jangala*, open grassy land, and *anupa*, marshy tree-filled land. A dry body was thought to come from eating meat raised on *jangala* land while a soft body (one given to fluxes) was thought to arise from eating meat raised on *anupa* land. The various Ayurvedic texts, treatises, and dictionaries catalog meats depending on whether they are *jangala* or *anupa*. This polarity is similar to the yin/yang polarity described previously from Chinese and Japanese medical practices (Trawick 1995: 282–284; Zimmerman 1982: 99–100). The medical polarity established by *jangala* and *anupa* allows treatments to be effected based on attempts to correct imbalance.

The notion of "wind" is also important. Ayurvedic texts describe a set of winds that move through the body such as breath (*prana*) and the wind that blows through the uterus, hollowing out the developing fetus. This wind (*vata*) is thought to animate the body and is one of three main substances. In addition, wind reflects climatic changes which bring alterations to the human body as it adjusts to seasonal variations. The other two substances are *pitta* (bile), which provides heat and luminosity to the body, and *kapha* (phlegm), which provides bodily moisture and cohesiveness (Trawick 1995: 284–285).

A central idea of Ayurvedic theory is that imbalance in one or another of these humors leads to illness. Thus treatment is directed at rebalancing disturbances that may result from within the body or from the social and environmental context in which the sick person is embedded. The Ayurvedic texts state that to diagnose disease the patient's signs and report of symptoms must be considered carefully rather than extensive physical examinations. Included in the texts are techniques for estimating temperature, smelling the breath, tasting the urine, and observing the patient so as to surmise the individual's caste. Treatment regimens include modifications in diet, exercise pattern, hygiene, and sleep. Natural medicinal mixtures composed of plants, minerals, and/or roots are used to rebalance the humoral system and restore health. In addition, heat treatment such as hot water or smoke may be used (Waxler-Morrison 1988: 532–533).

In the Ayurvedic texts the heart, *mahat*, is regarded as the seat of consciousness from which two sets of organs extend: the organs of action (hands, feet, mouth, and organs of generation and excretion), and the organs of sensation (eyes, ears, nose, tongue, and skin). All of the constructive substances of the body (*dhatus*) are thought to be joined to one another through a complicated set of synthetic actions in which one substance goes through a number of modifications until it is an end product. For example, food begins in the stomach and through this process is ultimately converted into a purified end product, such as semen (Trawick 1995: 285–286). This process is one of continuous conversion that can be equated with cooking in that one substance is converted into another through transformative steps that take place as substances move throughout the body. These conversions seem to be fueled by internal "fires."

As Zimmermann puts it, chyle, blood, flesh, fat, bone, marrow, and semen are transformed *in vivo* into one another by cooking. Growth of tissue as is seen as a result of consumption of food. Thus when a deficiency arises in the body a substance to offset it must have similar qualities to those of the deficient tissue. For example, in the case of a deficiency of semen, milk and clarified butter may be prescribed by the health care provider (Zimmermann 1982: 164–165).

The body is thought in Ayurvedic theory to be composed of specific channels through which each of the following separately flows: the three active forces (wind, bile, and phlegm), each of the senses, each of the constructive substances, and each of the waste products (*malas*). Disease is thought to arise when blockage of these channels occurs for whatever reason, thus producing an imbalance in the body as a whole (Trawick 1995: 286). We see from this account how a combination of notions regarding humors and their balance is the basis both for a theory of sickness and health and for a theory of what constitutes the human person. We have found the same in the other cases considered in this chapter. In the next chapter we turn to Papua New Guinea in order to look at what happens when fundamental ideas of this order interact with the introduction of biomedicine. We explore this theme partly through a discussion of a contemporary narrative of blood transfusion.

Chapter 3

Humoral Systems (2): The Melpa of Papua New Guinea

This chapter includes a case history of a narrative of blood transfusion from the Highlands of Papua New Guinea. An exploration of this case will provide the opportunity to discuss the question of what is in the blood from a number of viewpoints: how introduced medical practices are domesticated or transmuted in local understandings; how a single medical act is interpreted in collective and kinship terms; and how we can, from the narratives of the act, build up a picture of ideas about bodily substance that amount to a local theory of humors in the body and their connections with the identities and states of people.

The theoretical setting for this case study has to do with the conjuncture of two interests in anthropology: (1) changes in medical practices brought on by the introduction of biomedicine into contexts where ideas about sickness have stressed personalistic causal agency; and (2) the comparative study of humoral systems, which can be thought of as lying in between the impersonalities of biomedicine and the personifications found in forms of indigenous medicine, as in Papua New Guinea, for example.

Our starting point is the idea that there is indeed a fairly systematic set of ideas in the thinking of certain New Guinea peoples that we can reasonably label a humoral system and that regional variations are readily apparent.

To the Melpa speakers of Mount Hagen in the Western Highlands Province of Papua New Guinea blood may not be what it is in European popular traditions. Examining how it is and how it isn't is therefore a useful exercise in obtaining insight into indigenous ideas of sickness and healing. In European traditions, blood tends to stand for a generalized notion of kinship—consanguinity—that encompasses both agnatic and other ties in a general scheme of cognation or sharing birth origins. Among the Melpa, however, it tends to stand in a more specialized way for ties through females (although, Melpa usages are flexible and adjusted to certain real-world pragmatisms which cause blurring at the edges of this conceptual arrangement when it is convenient to equate rather than distinguish agnatic and other cognatic ties). Mother's kin, correspondingly, are thought to have special powers over the health of their nephews and nieces.

As outlined above (Ch. 2), in the Hippocratic humoral system there were four chief humors: blood, phlegm, black bile, and yellow bile, and these in turn were associated with human temperaments, seasonal sicknesses, and dietary practices. The guiding principles which steered Hippocratic medical ideas in relation to this scheme were (1) that the humors vary seasonally in their proportions in the body in terms of the axes hot/cold and wet/dry; and (2) that the all-important aim for health was to ensure balance and proper mixture between the elements. Food intakes, for example, could be used to maintain a proper constitution of the blood and to control too great an admixture of phlegm in the cold and wet conditions of winter that favored an unbalanced excess of phlegm.

As several commentators, (see Ch. 2), have remarked, when these Hippocratic ideas, transmitted into Hispanic culture via the Latin works of Galen, encountered indigenous notions in South America as a result of the Spanish conquest in the sixteenth century, the result was twofold: the seasonal correlations tended to drop out (not surprisingly since seasonal conditions are different in tropical from temperate zones), and the wet/dry component was downplayed in favor of the hot/cold distinction that seems, on the basis of most evidence, to have been indigenously established in many local cultures prior to Spanish contact.

The Melpa missed out on any direct historical encounter between their own classifications and European humoral notions, since they were introduced directly to biomedical ideas that have overlain humoral ones in western medicine. Their indigenous notions may be described as a two-humor rather than a four-humor system. The two humors are blood (*mema*) and grease (*kopong*), the latter comprising breast milk, semen, fat, the nurturant qualitiy in vegetable greens and other vegetable foods, and fertility in the soil itself. Although blood is not directly present in all the elements that have grease, red ocher, an earth product, is seen as like blood, and red-colored foods (such as the fruit pandanus, *Conoideus* sp.) are thought to help the blood or to replenish it. There is no idea that semen is concocted or purified blood as in the old European notion derived from Aristotle. Instead blood and grease form two separate but balanced and interconnected sources of vitality.

When this scheme is transposed into ideas of gender and kinship, we find that blood especially marks out ties through females. Agnatic ties (through males) may be referred to as "one penis" ties, and the notion here is that male semen is the constitutive element. Yet in both cases this clear division is modified: agnatic ties can also be referred to as "one blood," where blood stands for both blood and grease; and grease itself can refer equally to male semen and female breast milk. Blood and grease are a balanced gendered pair from one viewpoint, parallel and complementary (for example, they come together to produce a fetus, A. Strathern and P. J. Stewart 1998a), while from another viewpoint they each stand on both sides of the gender divide.

How do these two humors relate to ideas about health? In two ways. First, and of primary importance, is the idea of finite quantity. Both blood and grease can be "finished" in people, (or in the ground in the case of grease). There is in fact a considerable concern with either of the two humors being used up or finished in this way, because the end result is dryness rather than moisture, and dryness is linked with notions of aging, decay, and death. A man's grease is cumulatively used up in sexual intercourse and its depletion makes his skin dry and causes him to age; a woman's grease is used up similarly in feeding breast milk to her children. A woman's grease is also depleted through pregnancy. An old man fears that his blood is dry and finished; a woman experiences loss of blood in menstruation and is concerned that her blood will also be finished. Pork fat and juicy vegetables replenish grease in the body; red pandanus fruit and red-stemmed amaranthus greens replace blood. Either humor, if out of its proper place in time, can cause sickness: semen can spoil breast milk (hence the post-partum taboo on intercourse), and menstrual blood can harm men if ingested through the mouth or the penis (instead of causing fertility as it does when bound by semen in conception within the womb, it causes men's skin to dry up and ashes to rise in their necks, choking them to death, when it flows inappropriately in an external circuit).

Second, a triadic hot/cool/cold distinction applies. Blood that becomes too hot is "cooked" and dries up. "Cooking someone's blood" is a way of referring to hostile sorcery. Menstrual blood that is thought to have entered a man's body may be extracted in a number of ways, one of which is by applying sugarcane skins to the body surfaces and sucking at these, the blood then being spat out onto a heated drum lid in order to dry it up and destroy it. Heat, then, is associated with depletion, and sexual intercourse, which generates such heat, can dry up the grease of both sexes, as well as temporarily cook the blood. On the other hand, heat also indicates the presence of life, and cold its opposite, death. The optimal conditions for health and fertility are found in the balancing of hot and cold in the cool (*koma-tei*). For example, at the end of a cult performance when the sacred stones in the Female Spirit fertility cult were buried wrapped in moss and smeared with red ocher and white earth paints or pig fat they were said to be cool in this way (A. Strathern and P.J. Stewart 1997, 1998b, 1999b). Grease in the earth is cool; earth that is too hot loses its grease, and high mountain earth that experiences chilly rains and frost is also seen as either too dry or too cold to sustain life. The big-man, who leads a community, is supposed to have a mind or *noman* that is *koma-tei* also, avoid-

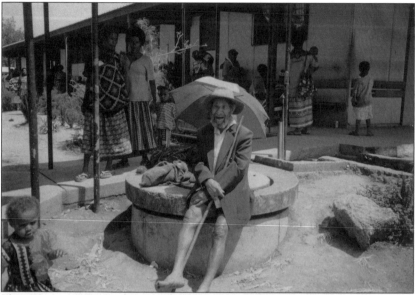

Figure 3–1. (1997) Ongka visits the Mount Hagen hospital to find out if his "blood is finished."

ing the heat of anger or *popokl*, and his actions that are sustained by his wives and others are supposed to make *kopong*, grease, for the group.

Does this humoral system interact with the system of ideas regarding emotions and sickness? Partially, certainly with respect to anger or frustration (*popokl*). *Popokl* is said to be experienced in the *noman* or mind/thoughts/ will, and the *noman* is not thought of as located in any single anatomical organ but generally within the sternum area. So it is not directly tied in with a body organ in this image. But it can also be said to be in the heart (*mundmong*), to make the heart rise up to the neck (blocking the normal exercise of the *noman* in speech), and to make fire to be in the heart (*mundmong ila ndip okla onom*). So, as in the lingua franca Tok Pisin term *bel as* (stomach hot), anger is understandably linked to heat, and it makes sense, therefore, that in general it connotes imbalance and a predisposition to sickness in the body of the person experiencing it. This point helps to explain why *popokl* is indeed thought to cause sickness not in others, but in the person who experiences it. The *noman*-based imagery is translated into the embodied imagery of heat and the heart to complete the causal chain. It is interesting, nevertheless, that the Melpa see the *noman* as the originary ethnolocation of anger, desire, envy, and other dangerous emotional states; while sympathy is said to be in the liver, and shame on the skin. The main point here is that the schema of balance is dominant throughout. Excess of anger causes sickness; excess of desire/envy leads to witchcraft; too much attachment or sympathy between a dead spouse and the living widow or widower can cause the ghost to come and take the survivor away; unbalanced acts lead to shame, which shows on the skin of people in blemishes or causes their skin to shake. Such an overall idea of balance clearly makes the Melpa humoral system comparable to others elsewhere. It is notable, also, that the two-humor system is itself a balanced one, and explicitly takes into account the reproductive side of life in terms of both blood and grease, whereas the four-humor Greco-European system does not give a place to a reproductive substance in its scheme, since this was considered in the corpus of knowledge controlled by females for the most part and set outside of the Hippocratic medicinal works on the whole (but see King 1998).

For the Melpa, conditions of health and sickness (by way of balance or imbalance between hot and cold) are present in blood; and blood signifies differences in maternal kinship and the power of mother's kin to influence sickness and health. What does not seem to be prominently coded in the blood, as it is in European folk ideas, is character. "Bad blood" can be a general synonym for "bad character" as when an elderly Kawelka male leader, Ongka, commenting on people's drinking habits, said that a person whose blood is bad (*mema kit morom*) becomes violent when drunk, whereas one whose blood is good (*mema kae morom*) merely becomes sleepy. But there is at present no evidence to indicate that this remark imputes an inherited or shared tendency within a collectivity, transmitted in some quality of blood. Rather, the remark seems to refer to a person whose blood is hot (and is therefore in a bad state) as opposed to one whose blood is cool (i.e. in a good, balanced state). These states could also be transitory and situational rather than stable over time. Character is most often located in the *noman* rather than in the blood/grease complex, and the *noman* is largely thought of as socially acquired. The basis for the development of pejorative associations of blood with character is thus missing, and this may help to explain why there is no great barrier to the acceptance of a new idea such as that of a blood transfusion among the Melpa. Blood means life, identity, kinship, collectivity, but does not appear to be predominantly linked with imputed character. Good blood is also on the whole blood that is balanced and flowing in its proper channels; the same with grease. And most significantly blood and grease are also finite, they may become scarce and be finished.

We suggest that for the Melpa blood and grease are elementary humors that are analogs or equivalents of wealth goods, such as pigs, shells, and money. Such a notion seems encoded in the principles of compensation for killings, as many writers have argued. Here we make this idea a bit more precise by arguing that it is the *humors* that are the analogs of wealth.

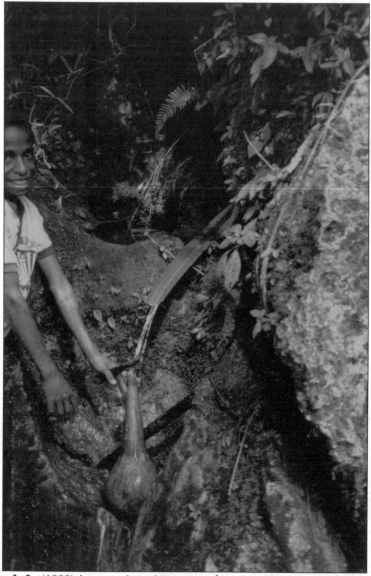

Figure 3–2. (1998) A mountain spring source of water at Hagu among the Duna. Water is an important "humoral" constituent of the body for the Duna.

There is evidence to support this view. For example, when blood is lost in an injury caused by an attack, the person who has lost blood says "replace/fix/fasten my blood" (*nanga mema pindi*), and what is meant is a demand for wealth to be given in compensation. Pigs, of course, are themselves amalgams of blood and grease, as well as bones, and they also have both *noman* (mind) and *min* (spirit) as humans do, so they are the closest analogs to humans. Shell valuables were sprinkled with red ocher, making them like an amalgam of blood (ocher) and grease (the shell itself with its whitish-yellow color). When money is given away in prestations it is adorned with red and yellow flowers and laid out on brightly colored lengths of fabric (A. Strathern and P.J. Stewart 1999a). Wealth goods are also expected to flow between exchange partners and kin, matching the implicit flows of blood and grease in creating kin relations, such as those deriving from females. If kin are dissatisfied with these flows, sickness results. The humors out of place are dangerous, like wealth that flows illicitly against body parts in order to pay for destructive magic made to kill people, or for assassins hired to strike people down directly with weapons. Wealth itself can be said to make grease between people: the term for friendship is the same as that for pig fat (*kng min*). Payments to maternal kin can be said to be made either for blood or for the "grease of the breast," i.e. mother's milk.

If, then, the overall idea here has some basis, we can suggest that gifts of wealth and gifts of blood could be equatable. The following case history will illustrate these points.

Ongka's Stroke

An aging leader among the Kawelka people in Hagen, Ongka-Kaepa, had a stroke in 1996 after suffering shock at the news of his son having struck a fellow sub-clansman and injuring him. He was taken to a hospital and eventually given blood transfusions. What follows is the narrative of his illness and ideas surrounding it, focusing on the novel transaction of giving blood.

One of Ongka's daughter's, Yara, explained what had brought on Ongka's stroke:

Yara

"Ongka became *popokl* [angry] because Kenny [a son of Ongka's] hit Kundil [a son of Rumba, a member of the same subclan as Ongka]. When Ongka heard the news of this he collapsed and was speechless and he got sick. People began to make prayers over him. Ongka is baptized in the

Catholic church and he is not supposed to get *popokl* over events or with people. They prayed, "Don't let him die, let him recover, let him not be *popokl*." [*Popokl*, as we have noted, is thought to make one sick and nowadays it is classified as an emotion that is sinful if not controlled.] After they prayed for him to be better they said that his heart was still beating and they took him to hospital. His blood was finished—there was no blood in him, the doctors said. He was first taken to Kotna health center [some twenty miles away] where they put a glucose drip feed into him. They looked for blood in his veins but there was no blood in them. My husband and I were looking after him there. Later, we decided to take him to the Hagen town hospital where they also gave him glucose and he began to get better. The hospital kept him overnight and the next day they gave him three packets of blood. The blood was from my daughter, Mopa, from Pekri and Mek, [two young men of a related Kawelka clan, the Membo], and from Nat, Ongka's sister's daughter. With the blood and the glucose Ongka began to get better because his blood began to work again."

In addition to the need for a transfusion Yara described how Ongka had a blockage in his throat that was preventing him from eating, improving, and being able to leave hospital for home:

"Ongka had blockages that were like saliva or spider's webs that were in his throat and these made him sick and would have killed him. I was looking after him and I had a bit of paper which I would use as these things came up into his mouth to wash and clean them away with a little water. The hospital staff saw me doing this and said not to do it. When they went away I continued to do it and eventually I removed all that stuff from his mouth. Then I went to the store and bought chocolate. I took this chocolate and made a prayer over it, saying "God, if it is your wish to take Ongka's life away, do that, but if it is your wish that he should live let me give him this chocolate and let it make some grease (*kopong*) in his throat and let him survive." At first when I gave him the chocolate it came back out of his throat so I mixed it with some water and let it drip slowly into his mouth and gradually I saw that it went down his throat and made some grease there—very slowly it went down, down into him—and after a while he began to move his fingers and move his toes and then I saw that he was coming back to life.

"Then I got some sweet bananas and I mashed them and started feeding them to him as one does to a little child, and after two days like this he gradually got better. Then the glucose drip was removed and he just took medicine to make him better. After one month Ongka left the hospital and went home. But when he was in the hospital he did not speak. He described when he wanted to urinate by using his fingers to signal to me and I would carry him on my back to the toilet. After returning home for three weeks he said nothing. Then he whispered for one week but we could not understand what he was saying—it was wild talk. We thought this was because he did not have enough food in him so we found pineapple and soft foods to give to him. Gradually then he started to speak, first like a child and then over time he got back his full powers of speech."

We asked Yara what the doctors had said Ongka's sickness was. She said, "Typhoid and malaria together—his blood was hot."

She went on to say:

"I thought to myself, my mother's dead and my brother's dead [i.e. Namba, the one son of Ongka who was said to have the potential talent and energy to succeed Ongka in the community as a leader] and now if my father dies what am I going to do? I tried to find some thoughts about this. I sought them and sought them but could find none. I could find nothing to do so I left it in the hands of God—God heard my prayers.

"All the relatives of Ongka of his blood, [*pundun kungan*, more remote relatives] had come and gave money, soap, or food while Ongka had been in the hospital but no officials of the Catholic church came to make prayers over him or visit him even though they knew he was in the hospital. I was the one to pray over him. There had been a collection of money for a coffin when Ongka was very ill but since he recovered one was not purchased. When Ongka does finally die he wants to be buried at Mbukl [his old settlement, twenty five miles to the north] near to where his son, Namba, is buried."

This ends the interview with Yara about Ongka's illness. She had said that he had no blood in his veins. What we ourselves were told when we took Ongka into the Hagen hospital for a follow-up exam was that he had anemia from malaria and needed to take iron tablets which we purchased for him. The doctors probably had tried to explain Ongka's anemia to Yara by using the Tok Pisin (lingua franca of Papua New Guinea) phrase, "em i no gat blus" which translates into "he does not have blood." After Ongka started taking his iron tablets following our purchase of them for him we noted a marked improvement in his energy level. The other medicine that we purchased for him after his examination was high blood pressure tablets (diuretics) which he also began taking but it was not clear to us how he would obtain additional medicine after our departure from the field area since he had no means of easily getting to the doctors for follow-up exams or to the chemists for refills on his prescriptions. We had left some money with Yara that was specifically for medicines but when Ongka heard that she had this money he demanded it be handed over to him for the collection of funds that he was putting together for a brideprice for another of his children, David.

Yara is devoted to her father. Her narrative of his illness depicts herself in the role of the mother taking care of the child. She gives him food like the sort that a child eats, feeding him chocolate which has a high fat content so as to coat his throat with *kopong* (grease) much as a mother pro-

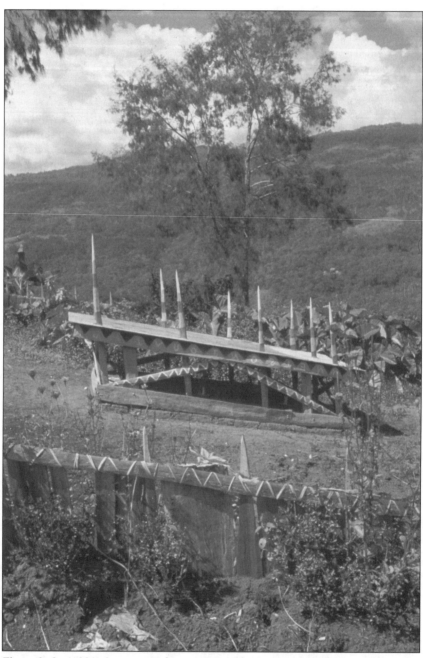

Figure 3–3. (1991) A ceremonial grave site at Aluni, among the Duna.

vides breast milk, a form of *kopong*, to her infant. Yara even found herself carrying Ongka on her back like an infant so that he could visit the toilet. She is seen to be a nurturing figure who corrects the imbalances in Ongka that are causing his sickness by providing him with the second humoral substance, *kopong*, after the blood transfusion had been given to rebalance the first humoral element.

Before Yara fed the *kopong*-containing chocolate to Ongka she made a prayer over it. This ritual blessing of the nurturing food helped to transform the commercially manufactured substance into something that was blessed by God.

Yara is an active member of the Assembly of God church and has carved out a niche for herself as a Christian dream interpreter and visionary. She described how prayers were made over Ongka before a heartbeat was found to still exist in him and how she prayed over Ongka and asked God to heal him if that was his wish to do so. Yara does not believe that the Catholic Church is the true church and she was highly critical of the fact that no Church official visited Ongka while he was in the hospital.

Ongka gave us his own account of the stroke:

Ongka

"There was a dispute between Kundil, the son of Rumba [a kinsman], and Kenny [Ongka's son] over some planks of wood that both men wanted. This took place in the market. Kundil hit Kenny over the head with one of the planks and Kenny took his bushknife and hit Kundil on the head causing him to fall over as if dead. The news came over to me from the market place as people called out from place to place relaying the news [this "bush telegraph" was a system used in the past as well as today to spread news of a killing] that Kundil was dead [the man did not actually die]. When I heard this the spirit went out of me. I had a shock! I said, "Why did he do that?" Then I collapsed and was taken to hospital.

"Immediately after I was taken to hospital the two sides involved exchanged pigs. One was sent over from Kundil's group for us to eat and my group sent a pig over for them to kill. This was done so that I wouldn't become too sick. I was unable to do anything myself. I didn't know anything about what was going on. It was done to try to stop my sickness from getting worse.

"Many people contributed money for my recovery—several hundreds of kina [one kina was approximately $0.50 in 1998]—so that I could eat special small foods like tins of fish and things like that. I ate these foods and gradually I got better. When I was sick they made prayers for me and asked God to give me three years more to live. To repay these people who helped me I took a very large pig of mine and I killed it and distributed it to them. The people did not want money in repayment so I gave this pig and distributed it out and said, "Eat it."

"That is how I got my shock—my own son struck down the son of someone who is like a brother to me, Rumba. This man, Kundil, did not die but an internal compensation of 10,000 Kina (approximately 5,000 USA dollars in May of 1998) was paid. I gave a couple of hundred kina towards this compensation payment. Also, five sets of eight pigs were given in the payment. I gave eight pigs, Kenny gave eight pigs, and others gave pigs to make forty pigs in all."

This ends Ongka's narrative of the event. He had on two separate occasions talked about his stroke, adding two additional points: (1) That the Kawelka had come together to donate blood for him—all the Kawelka he saw as being united in their efforts to help him recover, thus placing himself central in the political unification of the group as he has always seen himself to be. (2) That when prayers were made for his recovery it was asked that three years of life be granted to him after his recovery—one year of life for each day that he had been unconscious after the stroke. This three years for three days equation has a slightly Biblical air about it and we might speculate that Ongka sees his death occurring on the eve of the Millennium. Many Hageners declare that the year 2000 will bring the End Times to the world in the apocalyptic events depicted in the book of Revelations in the Bible (A. Strathern and P.J. Stewart 1997b; P.J. Stewart and A. Strathern 1998). Ongka has already asked that he be given a megaphone so that he can direct the people in their movements during the moments before the earth is destroyed in fire at the "End." Therefore, he must believe that he will be an important actor in this final show.

Two aspects of Yara's narrative that are notably absent from Ongka's are: (1) That he became *popokl*. He says that he had a shock, using the English word shock but not that he became *popokl*. In indigenous terms shock means that his *min* or spirit left him, leaving him as if dead, as he mentions. The word shock, he has clearly taken over from biomedical discourse. (2) He does not acknowledge the care that Yara specifically gave to him. He says that many people gave money and food to assist in his recovery but he does not name Yara as having cared for him in a special way.

Discussion

As we have seen, Yara's and Ongka's narratives overlap, but are different. Yara's narrative exemplifies most clearly the elements of the two-humor system and their intersection with the theory of *popokl*; also the intersection of all these notions with her appropriation of Christianity and

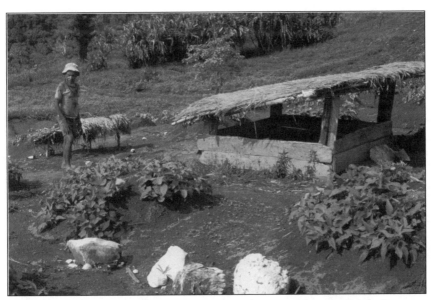

Figure 3–4. (1991) A regular grave site among the Duna. The "roof" is built so as to provide shelter for personal items that belonged to the deceased.

her emphasis on nurturing as an aspect of nursing. Both Ongka and Yara take pieces of information from an introduced world, of biomedicine on the one hand and Christianity on the other, and give these pieces meanings in their own terms.

The two-humor system of ideas shows quite clearly in the remarks that Ongka's blood was finished and that it was also hot because of malaria and typhoid; and in the notion that Ongka needed both blood tranfusions to replenish his own blood supply and the grease of the chocolate that Yara fed him. Indeed, the process is interesting. The blood was needed first because he could not live without it, and it was given on a personal and collective basis as well as on a professional basis by the hospital doctors. But in Yara's story her individual care and nurturance in feeding Ongka started him on the road back to his individual identity and his power of speech associated with his sense of that identity. She gives him back his identity by regrowing him from the state of an infant back to that of a man. Further, she does so as an individual and a daughter but also by invoking the will of God. The chocolate she gives becomes like a divinatory test of God's will, and she transforms it from a commercial object into a sacred one through her prayers, perhaps thereby aggregating it more closely to her own identity as a member of "the family of God" in the same way that food grown on clan ground imparts identity through its ancestrality of connection with clan ancestors (A. Strathern 1973). In any case, the doctors' actions are given meaning within the humoral system, and Yara gives to her own actions meaning both in terms of the idea of grease and its nurturing power and in terms of the combined agencies of herself and God.

In doing so Yara implicitly draws on an important sector of Hagen ideas linking food, nurturance, and identity all together. Identity as collectivity is given partly "in the blood," but it is also given by conscious acts of giving and sharing food grown on clan ground. Dyadic coidentity is also further expressed as a result of the optative choices of individuals in the practice of breaking a piece of food to share it and adopting the name of the food as a reciprocal name between the two persons involved in the sharing. Such food in turn is thought to build up the blood and grease in the body. Since blood is a transform of food, then the idea of a blood transfusion can easily be linked to notions of nurturance and identity.

This implies, however, that the blood should be particular blood, just as food should be particular food. Ongka received blood that was either from his "one blood" (*mema tenda*) kin as in the case of his daughter's daughter and his sister's daughter; or was from an affinal group, relatives of one of his wives, Ruk, of the Membo clan, and still within the general ambit of Kawelka identity. The transfusions combined cognatic, agnatic, and affinal values all together, contributing to Ongka's own view of himself as an icon of the Kawelka collectivity itself.

But, as we have already noted, Ongka himself stressed not so much the hospital transfusion as the balancing, public exchanges that were organized between himself and the kin of Kundil (whose blood was lost in the fight with Kenny) and in his act of cooking a pig for the people who contributed money to him for his subsistence while recovering from his illness. We may contrast here Yara's stress on her nurturing care (and the goodwill of God) with Ongka's own stress on the world of exchange as the fundamental locus of balance. Ongka's emphasis allows us to see the parallelism, however, between humoral theory and the theory of exchange: both depend on balanced flows. Ongka cannot directly repay a gift of blood with blood, but he does repay gifts of wealth with wealth, including pork grease for people to eat.

We see here also the overriding moral significance of the gift. Ongka feels he will not recover unless he morally rebalances his exchanges with others. The same emphasis on morality is seen in the idea of *popokl*, anger or frustration at other people's wrongdoing. The Christian religion has turned this around further, with the notion that it is the anger itself that is the wrongdoing, and what is important is to set one's exchange relationship with God to rights. Yara also invokes the primary context of morality when

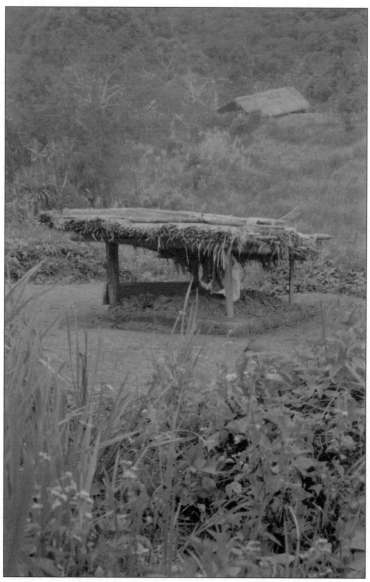

Figure 3 – 5. (1998) As 3-4; this picture shows a shirt hanging as a relic.

she effectively asks God to bless the chocolate she feeds to Ongka, invoking God, just as was done by invoking the ancestors and their effects on people's *noman* or minds in the pre-Christian system of thought and action.

What is in the blood from a Melpa point of view is a great deal of culture, history, and sociality particular to the contemporary context of life in Hagen. Blood has in it morality, the idea of exchange, nurturance, food, identity, collectivity, mortality, entropy, and finally a new possibility of transformation through the practice of transfusion, entirely novel to the Hageners, yet quickly given sets of meanings by the creative interpretive agency of those involved. Processes of interpretation and assimilation of this kind occur continuously on a daily basis in people's lives. They are the microcomponents of change and adjustment, often difficult to observe. A dramatic case history such as the present one allows us to detect and depict them a little more clearly: an analytical activity which is another version of seeing a world in a grain of sand—or in a package of blood.

These ideas about transfusion were gathered in 1997 prior to any local discussion of AIDS in our field area. By 1998 people were aware that AIDS exists and had begun to think about blood as a substance that could kill people as well as cure them. We expect to see these ideas developing rapidly as Papua New Guinea appears likely to enter into an AIDS-epidemic in the near future.

Melpa ideas are in many ways typical for the New Guinea Highlands region; however, their choice of the two humors blood and grease for emphasis in their practices can be seen as particular to them. In order to show that there are different arrangements of humoral ideas elsewhere we add here a sketch of the notions of the Duna people, who belong to Lake Kopiago in the Southern Highlands Province of Papua New Guinea.

The Duna

For the Duna people the humoral ideas of the body are expressed primarily in terms of three components: (1) blood; (2) other watery fluids; and (3) bone. We illustrate this briefly here from data on funeral practices.

The traditional platform burials and secondary burials focused on this two humor system. First the body of the dead person would be exposed on a platform structure suspended over a hole in the earth which had been dug in order to provide a receptacle for the "watery juices" that flowed out of the corpse during the period that it was exposed to the air for drying. These fluids were to be drained from the body and protected from consumption by animals. This practice is still observed in the current form of burial

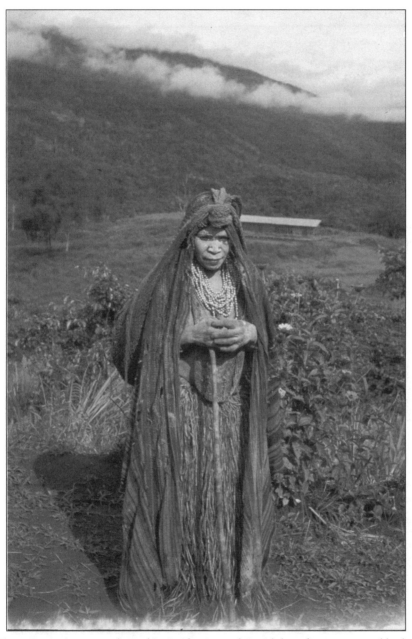

Figure 3–6. A woman dressed in "widow's weeds" with long front apron and body smeared with ashes and clay.

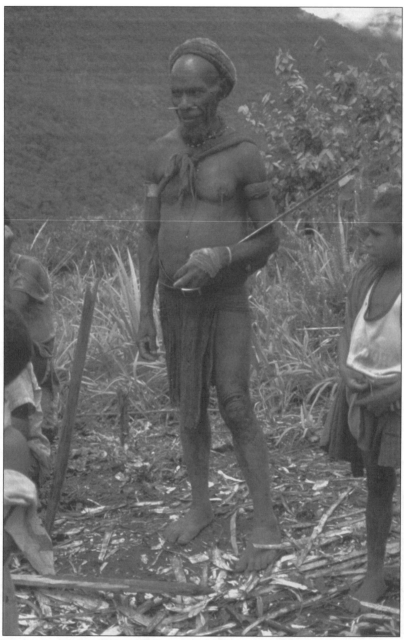

Figure 3–7. (1991) Wapiya, of Hagu Village, observes the preparations for constructing a grave site.

practices in which the platform burial is modified into essentially a submerged platform burial. Nowadays a body is buried in a deep grave inside of which a platform structure has been built and on this the coffin is placed. The coffin is provided with an opening through which the corpse's fluids drain out and are collected in the lower part of the grave underlying the platform.

In the past, after a corpse had been exposed for the requisite number of days on a platform, the remains (bones) of the corpse would be removed and placed in a cave which would serve as the burial vault and permanent repository for them. This site was considered to be the home for the spirit, *tini*, of the dead person and had to be taken care of by the kin of the deceased. If the bones of the deceased were disturbed by wild animals or not properly looked after in other ways the *tini* was thought to become disgruntled and send sickness to the neglectful kinsfolk, thus prompting them to go to the cave site and ensure that the bones were in order and undisturbed. Nowadays the Duna still believe that the home of the *tini* needs taking care of even though they do not always perform secondary burial, a practice which the Christian churches do not promote. Women sing special mourning songs to the *tini* of the deceased so that they will not be disturbed and angered thereby inflicting sickness or "trouble" on the living

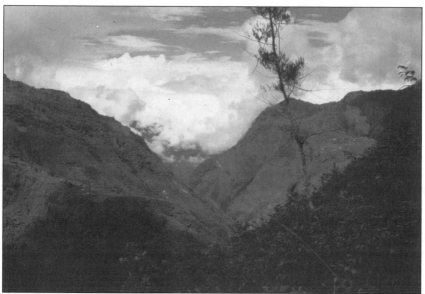

Figure 3–8. (1991) "Wild" country. The *tini* or spirits of newly dead people are told in funeral songs to depart into high mountainous areas like these.

relatives, and in particular to send them away to rock shelters in the forest like those where the bones are traditionally placed.

All of the Duna rituals that were focused on curing sickness or renewing the fertility of the ground (*rindi*) and its inhabitants used the blood of either humans or pigs. (In one story the pig is represented as having been in the mythical past buried on platforms and not eaten while human flesh was eaten and not properly buried: this story is discussed further in Ch. 5). Blood would be given to appease certain chthonic spirits (*tama*) and bring renewal. In addition, the bones of the ancestors had to be periodically fed in order to regenerate health and fertility. Chapter Five recounts some descriptions of these Duna ritual healing practices.

Chapter 4

Curers and Healers: The Melpa

This chapter continues the discussion in the previous chapter on the Mount Hagen area in Papua New Guinea, where indigenous specialists in medical practices, prior to the advent of biomedicine and Christianity, largely offered cures by the recitation of spells, which they had learned from other authorized practitioners. "Doctor-patient" communication thus largely consisted of the "doctor" talking to the spirit thought to have caused the sickness, or to the sickness itself, telling it to depart. Thus the treatment did not, on this view, treat the whole patient but rather the condition, as in biomedicine. On the other hand, sickness also could involve the whole patient because of the emotions in play and the belief that wrongdoing produces sickness. That is, the patient might be thought to have become ill because of wrong actions and the anger these had produced. In this case the specialist would sacrifice an animal (pig, marsupial) and invoke the patient's ancestors or ghosts in order to produce healing. A corpus of spells of the curing kind exists, but specialists could also be healers of the person, i.e., the guardians of their moral well-being.

We have made a distinction in this book between those who cure, *curers*, and those who heal, *healers* (see e.g. Introduction and Ch. 2). The former term is used to distinguish a person whose aim is to treat a physical ailment through attending to particular bodily malfunctioning. The latter refers to practitioners whose aim is to relieve illness caused specifically by immoral or improper actions. Of course, these terms overlap and intersect in most healthcare systems to some degree or another. We use the term *curator* here to refer to the holder of curative and/or healing knowledge. Sometimes these people are seen as practitioners while at other times, such as when Christianity condemns the use of these forms of knowledge, they are seen nowadays as repositories of "Satanic" knowledge (see also Brodwin 1996 on Haiti).

Some of the spells that ritual experts in Hagen used to employ in their curing practices are presented here. The term in the Hagen language for spell is *mön*. To show how these spells are supposed to work we give some examples.

Of the nine spells presented here 1, 3, and 4 are specifically spoken against spirit attacks; 2 consists of words spoken to accompany a divination designed to find the spirit responsible for a sickness; 5 is an antidote against a type of sorcery and 9 against the effects of menstrual blood thought by Hagen men to be dangerous to their health; 6, 7, and 8 are spells to help pigs grow. Experts spoke spells not only to deal with sicknesses but also to produce health and fertility, whether in humans or pigs. Whatever the specific purpose, the mode of imagery is similar throughout, creating pictures of actions taken to remove or block danger or of actions expressing health.

In the Hagen worldview the realm of the social/domestic (*mbo*) is contrasted with the wild asocial realm (*römi*). Wild spirits come from and must be sent back to their proper realm: caves, river junctions, stands of canegrass in swamps, and generally the wild low-lying valley area to the north of Hagen, known as the Jimi Valley, or the swampy banks of a large river, the Wahgi, that flows eastward from the central Hagen area.

Wild spirits, in the Hagen view, like to attack people, but they are able to do so only by invitation of the spirits of deceased kin. These are said to "open the fence" and let the wild spirits in (as wild pigs gain entrance to a garden by breaking through the fence) and to tell them whom to attack. In turn, dead kin do this only if they are aggrieved with their living kin or descendants for failing to care for them by giving sacrifices, or by separate wrongdoing such as in-group (as opposed to out-group) thieving, whether of property or of sexual access.

The spells image vividly two contrary movements: one of the movement of spirits along watercourses or through forests on their way to attack; and the other actions of the practitioner in driving them back to their caves, rocks, and riverbanks. Along with these two movements there are images of final actions: stilling a spirit's movements, pulling out a cassowary bird's pinions, setting up taboos against the spirit's return, imaging the recovered patient in terms of a Bird of Paradise with its healthy, glossy plumes or, again, a cassowary, known for its healthily voracious appetite.

The positive spells for fertility draw on ideas of rocks that stand out in flat country like the flanks of well-grown pigs, soft fertile ground, sprouting and multiplying seedlings, white wood of a tree, and bright soft stars as in the Milky Way. The expert does not posit a form of movement here but simply relies on an evocation of the process he wants to stimulate. Since these spells are said over pigs it is not supposed that the pigs understand them. If any extra-human agency is involved it is that of dead kin once more, favorably engaged as opposed to being punitive.

In terms of natural elements called on, it is notable that water is seen as a vector of power and a means of removing sickness. Spirits travel upriver to make trouble, going against the flow, and becoming "spirits out of place." They are sent back, with the flow, to their lower altitude abodes. Bespelled water itself is given to sick people to drink in order to flush the

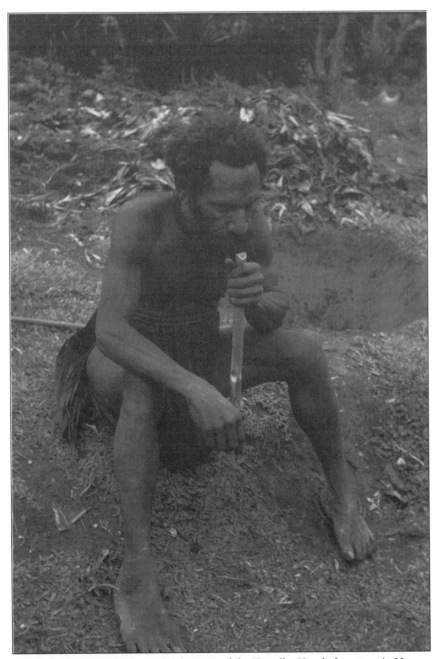

Figure 4–1. (1978) Moka, a ritual expert of the Kawelka Kundmbo group in Hagen, bespells water in a small bamboo tube before offering it to a patient to drink.

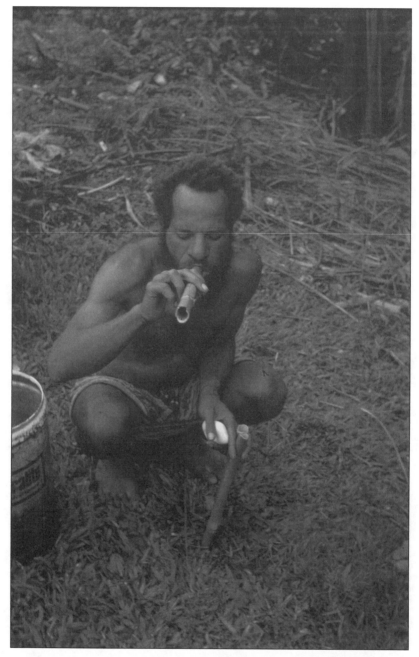

Figure 4–2. (1978) Nikint, Moka's nephew (elder brother's son) drinks the bespelled water.

poison of the sickness from their bodies and to direct it to flow away along the river courses also.

Spell # 2 represents the all-powerful image of the curer who controls the wild spirit that is causing the sickness. This action is like a targeted magic bullet that might knock out a cluster of cancerous cells.

Text of Spell 2

> At the Ukl stone, at the Mangka stone,
> Where the Antep shrub stands up straight,
> I pull out the pinions of the wild cassowary,
> I still the movements of the two *kumbaem* marsupials,
> I bring it down to the base of the mountain beech,
> I fasten it down,
> I pull out the pinions of the wild cassowary.

Texts from the other spells (1, 3–9) are as follows:

1. *A spell to drive away a wild spirit*
   At the banks of the Wahgi, banks of the Gumant,
   Where a clump of ferns is growing,
   It comes, peering up, looking around.
   The spirits of dead kin have opened the fence,
   And now the wild spirit comes.
   Let it go back to the places in the east it comes from.

3. *A spell against a wild spirit*
   An Antep shrub grows tall.
   The Ukl stone stands up.
   Quietly it comes, looking out.
   "Should I go this way or that?"
   And then it sees
   Our mother, father, brother, son,
   Daughter, those who are dead,
   Signal to it, beckoning.
   "I told them to give me
   The big sow, the big barrow pig,
   But they refused,
   So now you strike them for me,
   Try and see what you can do."
   "Truly?", it says, and "Truly, yes!"

   They say.....
   So it goes secretly and strikes,
   And the sick person sacrifices a pig.

"Alright, now you can go,
I place you back on the Ukl stone."

4. *A spell against "small spirits" that attack. Note: these also may bring good luck. They are spirits that are like children.*
At the junction of the big rivers Baiyer and Möka
It builds its many-coloured house.
On the banks of the Möka it takes the flower of
      the cane grass plant,
It takes the flower of the Membokl banana,
It takes the flower of the Keninga banana,
At the banks of the Möka, the banks of the Angekl;
Along the Ombil, along the Embö,
Along the Ropöng, along the Mbakla,
Along the Yanga, walking unsteadily,
Walking firmly, wearing
A single plume of the White Bird of Paradise,
Wearing a headnet painted with red ocher,
It comes, it comes along, until
The dead spirit opens the fence to it,
And so it comes inside, wild as it is.
"Now you go back to the river junctions
Where you live, now I have made
A sacrifice of a red and black pig,
Now I put you back
Down by the river junction where you belong."

5. *An "antidote" spell* (against the form of sorcery known as *kundumou*, where a piece of pork fat is cooked to attract the spirit of a victim and the spirit is lured into a hole and packed into it, to die there. In the antidote the expert uses a cassowary leg-bone dagger to dig up the soul and release it and to send the bad power away).

He fought, he killed,
And for that they did this, I see.
I take it and put it back with the wild fowl,
With the *klomanda* bird,
I clean it out and take it away,
Place it where the two rivers join.
It calls out as the bird of bad omen,
I strike it with a burning piece of wood.
It calls out and goes off to the Rauna river,
Down in the wilderness of cane grass

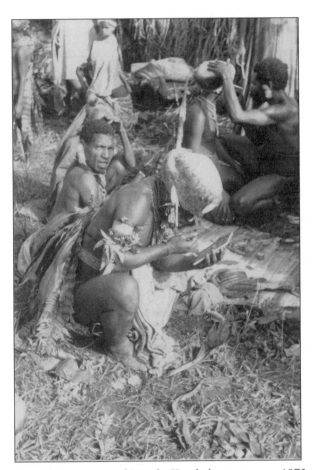

Figure 4–3. Eip, a woman married into the Kundmbo group, at a 1973 preparatory occasion for the Female Spirit cult. Eip is a ritual expert, who in her spells calls on the mountains Ialibu and Giluwe to help pigs grow. She is looking at the camera, with a tuft of marsupial fur in her ear.

I take it there and put it where the two rivers join.
The *mara* leaf stands up at the Möka's edge,
The *kengena* leaf stands up at the Baiyer's edge.

The sorcery is personified and seen as being driven away like a wild spirit.
The leaves "stand up" forbidding its return, or else marking the return of
the patient's health.

6. *A spell to make a sow be big*
At Ep, At Ambra,
The hill stands out.
Garden soil filled with soft roots
Springs up beneath the foot.

The pig's body should stand out as these hills do from the plain. Its flesh
should be full and spring back like fertile soil underfoot.

7. *A spell to make a pig's litter grow fast*
The amaranth seedlings multiply and grow,
The cucumber seedlings multiply and grow,
The lagenaria seedlings multiply and grow.

All these plants are known for their ability to grow swiftly and in large
numbers.

8. *A spell to increase the layers of fat in the skin of pigs*
Like the Mimb lake, soft, soft.
Like stars in the Milky Way, soft, soft.
Like the round rock Mbane at Ambra,
Like the two stones with shining heads,
          Pon and An,
Like the small stars that melt away at dawn,
Like the Poembukla tree, whose bark reveals
White flesh beneath —
Like this you will be.

9. *A spell against the effects of contact with menstrual blood*
("A woman has slept in the menstrual hut and put on us the
sweat from her armpit, she has transmitted the dirt from her
hands, she has stepped over us, why we do not know, the blood
flows, so now....)
I fill up water from the Mbakla and give it,
I fill up water from the Ombil and give it,
I fill up water from the Yanga and give it,
I fill up water from the Kauklorong and give it,

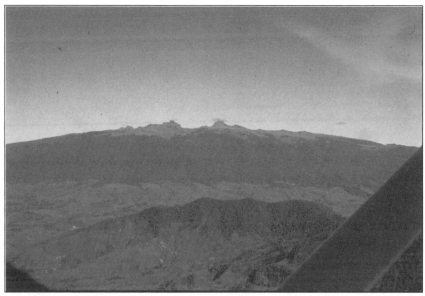

Figure 4–4. The mountain Giluwe, south of Hagen, a focus of images in spells (see spell no. 9).

I fill up water from the Eimbo and give it.
I fill up water and pour it in,
I make it flow and take it away,
Away, away, down where the Möka and Anggekl
        rivers meet,
Where the black tail-plumes of the Sicklebill
        Bird of Paradise stand up firm,
Where the wild cassowary grunts eagerly over
        its food,
Where the flying fox from Giluwe regurgitates
        its refuse.

[The three images at the end represent the patient's recovered health: his skin will be glossy like the bird's feathers, he will have a healthy appetite like the cassowary, and he will get rid of the blood as the flying fox vomits up its refuse.]

(All these spells were recited by the ritual specialist Mambogla of the Kawelka Kundmbo group, 10/11/65. They were translated from the Melpa language 12/05/97.)

Discussion

Medical anthropologists have used various ideas to bring into conspectus the practices of curers and healers around the world. It is commonplace to observe the marked differences between biomedicine and other systems, while it is also feasible to establish cross-cultural similarities. In all systems there is a need for an at least partly shared framework of ideas between patients and practitioners. However, it is common to find divergences and disparities of knowledge, simply because the practitioner is the specialist. Communication is based on the shared aspects of such a framework, enabling patients to accept diagnoses and treatments.

In an article entitled "Sacred Healing and Biomedicine Compared," Finkler has commented that comparisons between biomedical physicians and folk healers sometimes take an evaluative form. In one view folk healers are romanticized and described as having an ideal relationship to the patients. In the other, contrary, view folk healers are dismissed as charlatans who impede the work of physicians (Finkler 1994b: 179). She points out the inaccuracies of both views and enters a more extended discussion based on Mexican Spiritualist healing versus biomedical practice (see Ch. 7). Here we are also concerned with similarities and differences not centered on imputed *efficacies*, but on perceived *logics*.

First, the logic of biomedicine implies that the aim of diagnosis is to establish a condition, its causes, and therefore its treatment, especially with regard to its cure or its alleviation. The focus is material, on the body, and on techniques and tools of examination, and the chief aim is to find pathogens and/or degenerative processes. Communication with the patient and examination of the patient's body is undertaken with the above aims. In the logic of the spells we have looked at here the condition of the patient's body is taken for granted: the patient is ill. Sometimes if one asks of the patient "Well, what sickness does he/she have? (*elim namba kui ti ronom?*)" there is a puzzled response from kin: "Well, it is just true sickness! (*kui ingk ronom-eka*)." The expert's insight and communicative effort are engaged with the spirit entities involved, and both diagnosis and cure are contained in the spell narrative and its imagery.

Second, in accordance with the communicative focus, it is assumed that the patient will recover if the wild spirit departs and the domestic spirit is appeased by a pork sacrifice. The domestic spirit receives the sacrifice, enjoying its "smell." The wild spirit is just told to go away, politely but firmly. The focus is therefore on personalistic agencies, not on naturalistic causes. This focus does not, however, mean that people avoid the introduced biomedical system with its reliance on the idea of naturalistic causes. As everywhere, people are pragmatic and will use anything that seems to work.

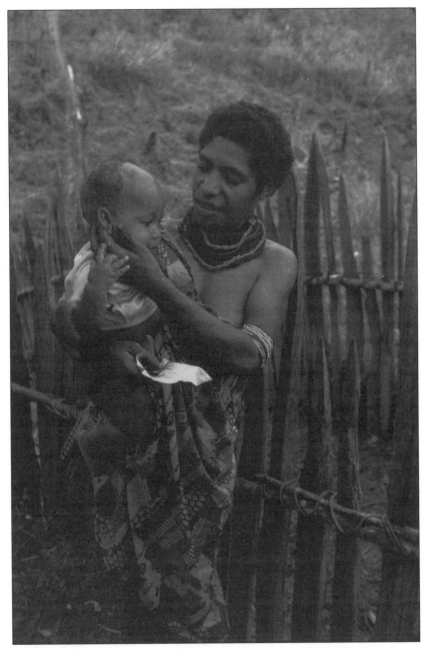

Figure 4-5. The wife of a Kundmbo man, Wömndi, whose child was suffering from cephalic scabies and also received treatment from Moka. Yellow mud was plastered on the child's head.

Third, the sick person and the kinsfolk do not hear the exact words of the spell because these are muttered or whispered to the spirits involved. But the patient and kin do know the framework because this has been explained to them in advance and they are familiar with it. This framework also implies a moral situation if the patient or kin reveal some wrongdoing as the possible cause of the sickness.

Fourth, the spell narrative also encapsulates the manipulation of the symbolic framework. Action is taken: the spirit is sent back. The spell thus functions as both diagnosis and cure. It is as though a physician looking into a microscope observed a pathogen, said so, and at the same time removed it by saying that this was what she or he was doing. The functions variously distributed in diagnosis, prescription, and cure in biomedical practice are thus all packaged into the spell plus the accompanying actions that often take place, e.g. smearing the patient's body with cooling clay or giving the patient water to drink from bamboo tubes. These accompanying actions and the items used in them, *tamb-mel*, form another bridge to biomedicine, since *tamb-mel* are like medicines, and may also be used without spells, as leaf irritants are used to relieve pain by counteraction.

In a peri-urban area some twenty-five miles nearer to the town than the home of the practitioner who recounted spells 1–9, a specialist was interviewed who declared that his forte was also in removing wild spirits. This specialist, however, had already made an accommodation with change. About a mile from his home place, Keluwa, was the Lutheran Mission station Ogelbeng, established in the 1930s. Many people were already baptized by 1964, and this mission forbade people to use indigenous magic. The practitioner, Pombora, declared that he knew this and therefore had cut out the use of spells but retained the accompanying actions. His main technique had to do with sexual attacks on women by wild spirits, making them pseudopregnant. He would rub the abdomen of a woman so affected with the leaves of a fine type of indigenous cooking banana and call the wild spirit inside to come out and leave the woman's body. In exercising power like this he was in fact helped by a wild spirit whom he had tamed and adopted by offering it a sacrifice of pork in a small cult house. It came in the form of a snake and licked his face and hand, and his power was said to come from the snake's smell on his hand. Pombora's version of "healing touch" thus depended on the idea of smell and spirit residue. Second, Pombora claimed to have made an accommodation with biomedicine and with white people's ideas. He reported that there was a wild spirit that used to attack the cows of a white man and also attacked him, in the guise of a female. A cow died, and Pombora was called in and paid five pounds [the Australian currency then in use] for getting rid of the spirit. Finally, he claimed that he could be called in to help in difficult cases by the Australian physicians in the town hospital when women were suffering from pseudopregnancies caused by spirit attack. Pombora thus self-hybridized and self-bracketed his activities, with the aim of portraying his skills as legitimate and useful in both the indigenous and the introduced worlds of practice. His assertions are to be seen as a halfway house to the takeover of pragmatic curing by biomedicine. Biomedicine, however, cannot effectively deal with entities outside its framework, such as wild spirits, ghosts, and witchcraft. The churches can do so to some extent, through exorcisms and protective prayers that function as spells do. They can also deal with moral issues by asking people to confess wrongdoing and/or anger and call to God for forgiveness and removal of sickness brought on by these means. The churches today have substantially taken over the healing functions met in the past by sacrifices to appease dead kin.

Many things have changed since the 1960s. Aid posts (local facilities that provide limited services such as dispensing aspirins and medicine for conditions including leprosy or malaria, giving penicillin injections, and treating minor wounds) were established and subsidized by the government. The services at these posts were provided by persons who had received one to two years of basic training in medical practices and who were given a small wage. These aid post attendants were also supposed to receive payment for their services from their patients in the form of food, firewood, or money. In addition to aid posts, hospitals were introduced in the urban areas. These were — and are today — heavily subsidized by the government. During our field visit to Hagen in 1997 we found that aid posts were largely inoperative and public hospitals grossly overcrowded.

The beginning stages of severe drought brought on by El Niño-induced climatic changes were starting to cause food shortages by mid-1997 as crops were failing. The drought continued into early 1998. Famine conditions existed and government relief foods such as rice and flour were brought in. The diseases such as malaria, typhoid, and dysentery that generally plague the region were killing more people because they were in a weakened state.

Two ideas increasingly prevalent among the local people that are used as devices to cope with the uncertainty of the times are (1) notions that witches are more abundant and that they are making people sick in addition to killing and eating them (P.J. Stewart and A. Strathern 1997); and (2) millennarian ideas of the World's End, in which it is thought that shortly Jesus will return to the earth and the "faithful" will be saved from the destruction which will consume the followers of the Antichrist (P.J. Stewart and A. Strathern 1997b; 1998). Some people have also, perforce, turned again to indigenous forms of medicine to ease their suffering, since Aid Post medicines are not available to them.

In principle, then, biomedicine takes over the curing functions of indigenous practitioners with prescriptions (words) and applications of substances (treatments). The churches take over healing functions by reintroducing the moral element into the removal of sickness. The traditional practitioner's dual curing/healing functions are thus split up. Indigenous curing re-emerges when state medicinal services do not adequately meet the needs of the populace, while Christianity has continued to take on the role of the healer through its moral guidance.

One of the traditional causes of sickness is *popokl* (anger/frustration) directed against someone who has acted in a way that is thought to be unjust. The person who experiences *popokl* becomes ill and the person who is the source of the frustration must be found and made to alleviate the sick person's *popokl* in order for recovery to begin. Nowadays the church teaches that *popokl* itself is a sin and that those who become sick from *popokl* are acting immorally and reducing their likelihood for entrance into Heaven. The churches thus deal with one part of the moral spectrum but not with the other. They ask the angry person to forgive the wrongdoer rather than demanding compensation or seeking revenge.

Another way in which the church is attempting to control health through moral guidance is by condemning sexual promiscuity. AIDS and other sexually transmitted diseases have become an increasing health problem in PNG over the last decade. Both male and female prostitution have hastened the spread of these diseases.

The concept in Hagen of *mön*, ritual practice, encompassed a range of functions of both curing and healing, all bound up in the idea of the spell. The practitioners of this healing or curing were well esteemed and paid rather generously for their services. Their practices came under attack from both hospital clinicians and missionaries, who have between them reparceled out the functions of *mön* in different directions. From our point of view as anthropologists, a textual analysis of spells shows that they conform to the most general model of medical practice: diagnosis and treatment, informed by a more or less shared symbolic framework and action taken within it.

Among the Duna people, whose humoral ideas we have glanced at briefly at the end of chapter three, there was an extremely elaborate panoply of rituals aimed at dealing with sickness in a cosmic framework. We devote the next chapter to a discussion of some of these Duna rituals and their drastic curtailment as a result of religious change and the introduction of biomedical practices.

Chapter 5

Duna Ritual
Practices and Healing

The Duna people live far to the west of the Melpa in a remote corner of the Southern Highlands Province of Papua New Guinea. Like the Melpa, they are intensive horticulturalists depending on the sweet potato as their staple and rearing pigs for use in sacrifices, life-cycle payments, and indemnifications for injury or killing. They live in bounded social areas that are clearly named and called parishes in the ethnographic literature. The parishes consist of a conglomerate of kinsfolk and associates, some migrants from elsewhere. They are centered on a small core of patrilineal members known as *anoagaro*, who traditionally have positions of command over leadership, land, and ritual knowledge in the community. Parishes were engaged in warfare with each other up to the 1960s when Australian colonial control reached the area following isolated earlier patrols. The area overall has experienced very little economic development by comparison with Hagen, although a minimal infrastructure of roads, schools, and aid posts (often not well stocked) exists. The influence of Christian missions (Catholic, Seventh Day Adventist, Baptist, and Apostolic in particular) has been marked, and most people are nominally Christian. The rituals we discuss here have on the whole not been practiced since the 1960s when missions first arrived, although since 1996 there has been a revival of antiwitchcraft procedures which we discuss. Aid Post medicines have been adopted readily, but at a deeper level old ideas remain, although metamorphosed.

The Duna people have historically been deeply concerned with the fertility of the earth seen as a single cosmos and have ritually attempted to stave off an anticipated world's end some fourteen generations after the putative founding of the patrilineal lines in the parishes. Rituals to maintain the cosmos and restore it to health were called *rindi kiniya*, "straightening/remaking the ground." Signs of the earth's decline were crop failures, droughts, infertility of women, poor growth in plants, animals, and children, and general sickness. Nearly every major and many minor rituals were tied into the goal of maintaining the cosmos. Curing sickness was a part of this process of maintenance and renewal. Such curings were simultaneously healings, contributing to the welfare of the wider whole. These powers of healing were opposed by those of witchcraft, which we deal with in sections one and four below.

To give the reader an idea of primary ethnographic materials, this chapter provides some partial transcripts of interviews about the 'old days' when healing rituals were performed. We follow these with a discussion of changes since then. All of the informants were highly knowledgeable senior men who acquired their knowledge from their fathers and their own observations. They volunteered their narratives in response to general requests for indigenous knowledge in various spheres. A great many narratives turned on questions of ritual, sickness, growth, health, and fertility, showing these to be major concerns. Today's male pastors are often former ritual experts who have deliberately withheld transmission of their knowledge since becoming Christian pastors.

[We translated the following ethnographic materials from Tok Pisin (the lingua franca of Papua New Guinea) and have paraphrased the translations in this chapter for clarity of exposition.]

1. Ideas of Witchcraft

An elaborate set of ideas surrounds the notions of witchcraft. Many ideas are explained in a myth about its origins.

The story of the origin of witchcraft was told to us by an expert informant and local Government Councillor, Mr. K.-H., in 1998 (Stewart and Strathern 1998) and goes as follows:

"Witchcraft arose in the village of Yeru [at the Strickland river which marks a boundary of Duna territory]. It came up from a place where there is a little hole in the ground. From this hole a witchcraft spirit man, *tsuwake tama*, came forth. This happened during a time when the people were killing pigs, making houses, and preparing earth ovens for cooking [probably referring to preparations made during one of the rituals in which sacrifices to the earth were made to prolong its fertility]. This spirit man came up and stood upon a stone. This stone is still standing today and can be seen by people who pass by it.

"This spirit man just stood upon the stone and all the men who were dancing around [as part of the ritual performance] saw him. He began eating the heads of the men and throwing their bodies aside... Then a woman passed by the place and the *tama* wanted to kill her but the woman said to him, 'Let's be friends—don't kill me.' The *tama* agreed and they stayed together. The woman then had two children, one girl and one boy. Subsequently she gave birth to many, many children. They did not eat pork but ate human flesh. They buried pigs when they died and at that

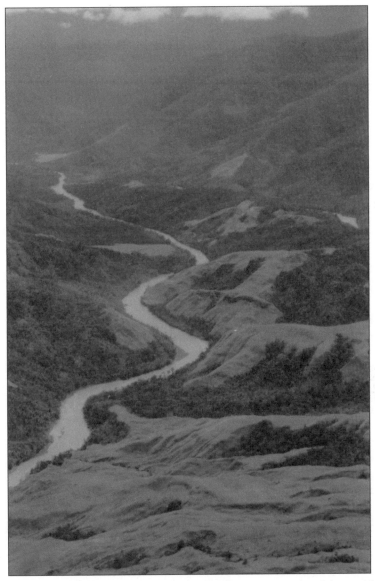

Figure 5–1. Grassland and forest at the Strickland river gorge, site of the mythical origin of witchcraft among the Duna.

time especially they killed a human and ate it. Both the men and the women were cannibals.

"A man from Koroba [south of the Duna area] called Hambua was carrying salt with him and was travelling along the 'road of the leg of the pig' [this probably refers to a ritual trackway in which sacred sites were marked out and performances to renew the earth were enacted. At the end of this trackway was a spirit who lived in a hole and was given sacrificial offerings on a periodic basis in order to ensure the fertility of the earth (A. Strathern and P.J. Stewart 1998; P.J. Stewart 1998; P.J. Stewart and A. Strathern n.d.)].

"He came along and found that a pig that had died was being prepared to be buried and that an earth oven had been made in which a woman was going to be cooked. All of the people had gone to collect materials (firewood and vegetable greens) for the cooking. The woman who was going to be killed and cooked remained at the cooking site. Hambua asked the woman if there was going to be a pig cooking. She said, 'No, they are going to eat me.' 'But what about the pig there?' Hambua asked. 'Oh, it just died.' The woman began to cry but Hambua said, 'Don't do that. This pig can be eaten. You are a human and should not be eaten.' He and the woman cooked the pig and when the people came back they smelt the odour of the cooked pork and said, 'This is a bad smell, of a dead body.' But Hambua had his salt and he told them to eat the pork with salt on it and that it was good that way. The people did eat the pork and were then instructed to kill pigs and eat them but not to kill and eat humans.

"The offspring of the original male *tama* and the woman he found and decided not to eat were mixed; some were animal children—snakes, cassowaries, and marsupials, some were true human children and these were the ones that were shown to the public. The animal children were witchcraft familiars and their mothers kept these inside themselves."

In 1991 K.-H. [this informant has been referred to by the pseudonym of Karua elsewhere] also provided an interview. Andrew Strathern asked him a set of questions, the answers to which further elaborate some of the points made above.

"*Tsuwake kono* is a type of witchcraft that women have. Wild animals come up in them such as wild pigs, cats, cassowaries, and marsupials. Only a few women have this. I look at these women and I know which ones have it. They kill men and they steam cook them at the lakes known as Ipa Ane such as Alu lake.... They have meetings and they come together to eat at these pools of water where the victim is killed and eaten while all of them watch. Mothers teach their daughters these things...

In the past there were good men and bad men. It was a bad man who taught witchcraft to women...A witch knows when you are sleeping. At the time of sleeping the *tini* (spirit) goes out of the body and it returns when he awakens. A witch sees the *tini* of a person coming out of his body and kills it and the person later dies because of this. But the witch doesn't cook and eat the victim quickly; rather the *tini* of the victim is placed in a tree during which time the person gets sick with headaches or back pain and only later actually dies. There is no medicine to stop this. If a person were just sick medicine could help cure them but if a person is ill from witchcraft then medicine will not work. In the past a male ritual expert could use a divining stick (*ndele rowa*) to detect witchcraft. A few men still have this knowledge... The *ndele rowa* follows witches, leading the diviner to the house of a female where items such as a bamboo knife, vegetable greens, cooking stones [used for an earth oven] and bones from the victim, will be found... Alu Sisa was a man who could use the *ndele rowa* because he was with the Payame Ima [the Female Spirit who gives men the power to divine for witchcraft]... The Payame Ima protected Alu Sisa..." [the interview goes on with K.-H. stating that witchcraft was first derived from the male *tama* spirit that he spoke of in the lengthier interview provided above].

We will see the relevance of this origin story today in the narrative on events of witchcraft in 1998 (sect. 4 of this Ch.)

2. Male and Female Ritual Experts

a. Story of How a Male and Female Ritual Expert Worked to Cure Sickness. Au of Nauwa Parish (Sept. 10, 1991)

"I will tell a story of how a father's sister of mine performed curing magic. They did this when people felt pain in their bodies. A special kind of ground/clay was rubbed on their skin. The sick person might be suffering from malaria and feel pain and thus might visit this curer. There was a male expert involved also, he would rub ground on the skin of the sick person. The female expert would ask the sick person what was wrong with them, if their skin felt hot or if something else was wrong. Then the sick person would reply, saying for example, 'my skin is hot and painful.'

"The male expert would say, 'I will go and find leaves from the *towa andi* tree and from the *kapiruku* fern plant. These leaves have a sweet odor like that from marsupials [various marsupial species are hunted and eaten in this area of Papua New Guinea]. The expert would lay the leaves out separately and bring yellow (*hambua*) colored ground to place on top of the leaves. On top of this he would pour water. The expert would then take

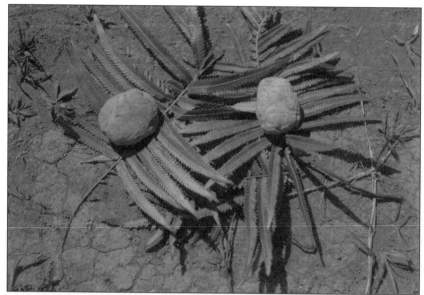

Figure 5–2. Yellow (*hambua*) and white (*kiapo*) types of clay used in ritual healing (Duna).

the ground and apply it to the skin of the sick man, starting at the upper part of the body and working downwards towards the feet. The leaves that had been used were not thrown away but were kept carefully. When the patient was covered with the *hambua* ground he was told to sleep during the night: 'This ground whose specific name is *tambo rindi* will help you sleep.'

"If the patient slept alright, the next day the expert rubbed his body again with *tambo rindi*. The next morning the sick person would be asked if he slept alright and if so then on the following day the coating of mud that had been applied to his body would be removed.

"This procedure was for heat on the skin. The male expert dealt with this. The female expert dealt with pain which I will describe next. Both of these experts were paid with cowrie shells [cowrie shells were one of the main forms of traditional wealth in the past before money entered into this part of the world.]

"The female expert would go to the area where the patient lived. Many people from Aluni parish [one of the main villages within the Duna area where we conduct our research] would consult her [Au is describing his aunt who was a female ritual expert]. She would ask what the problem was with the person, and ask that the type of pain that they were experiencing be described, e.g., in the knee or the back. These people with pain would not sleep well at night and this was also one of their complaints.

"This female expert brought with her a special type of earth, *kiapo rindi* (white clay) [This type of earth was used in other ritual practices that stretched out across the landscape through ritual trackways, thus we see here this earth being used in practices that aim to 'renew' the earth and also in curing rituals]. *Kiapo rindi* is the general name for this type of earth. The name of the particular kind used in this ritual was *sope sope*. This earth would be put onto a *payeku* (type of cordyline) leaf and the leaf and earth were then examined to determine if any stones or hard objects were affixed to them. If not, then water was poured over them. Next, the curer would rub the ground on the sick person's skin, holding the earth in place and then rubbing again repeatedly while moving along the person's body until an object was discovered to have come out of the body of the sick person. This could be a chip of flint (to cut the insides), a stone (to make the skin turn black [perhaps as in a bruise], a piece of sharp bamboo (also to cut the insides), a clump of marsupial fur, tree moss, or fireplace ashes/charcoal.

"The people who were gathered around to observe the ritual procedure would ask, 'What is it that you have found?' The expert would reply, 'This moss belongs to the *Payame Ima*" [a Female Spirit category in the Duna area who provides male ritual experts with the knowledge to divine who are witches in the community and have produced sickness in a person, see section 1 above]. This was hidden in the bush in trees. The *Payame Ima* put it there. She would say, 'If you go hunting in the bush with your dog and hear a sound and see a hole of the *wii yukilini* marsupial [one of the manifestations of the *Payame Ima*] you will know that it is this that has held you with its hand'.

"As for the fireplace ashes/charcoal, she would say, 'This means that when you kill a pig you must color the killing club with this residue which is red.' [The color of red symbolizes the father's side of the sick person while the color black symbolizes the mother's side]. The expert would take *towa sondo* (ashes) and put them on a leaf and ask that they be placed by a *tale* tree [a tree that is associated with the *Payame Ima*]. Then earth would be put on top of this leaf and the expert would say, 'Apapa Apapa, Apapa, (Mother's side, mother's side, mother's side), Auapa, Auapa, Auapa (father's side, father's side, father's side)...,' in order to divine which side of the sick person's family was causing the sickness.

"After determining this they would make two small holes in the ground that would serve as receptacles for the blood that would flow from the nose of a sacrificed pig. One pig was killed in the women's house and cooked there. The ashes/charcoal that had been removed from the patient's body by the expert would be rubbed onto the nose of the pig. Since it had been determined that on this occasion the person's sickness had been produced by the kin on the father's side, a large pig was killed, and was called *tama kuma* (spirit nose). The pig was killed in a special way with a stick that had red and black paint on it, [representing the two sides of the patient's family]. All of the kinsfolk of the patient came together on this occasion.

"The expert would take leaves from cordyline, fern, and taro plants and plant these and place them in three holes and cover these with black stones. The female expert told all the people to come and watch as she called all the ghostly kin involved to come and sit on the stick used to kill the pig. She took the stick and hit the pig and the head of the pig was then lifted and placed in the hole to collect its blood while its legs were held in the air. She would say that whichever kin were involved in making this person sick they should take the sacrifice of the pig and go. She would refer to whatever specific type of pig it was that was being sacrificed, e.g. its color or its skin pattern. Then the pig would be removed from the hole and cooked that night...People would look into the hole at the blood of the pig for a sign of who had actually produced the sickness. The expert would look for a *kalongane* (an omen). If there was a bit of vegetable greens in the blood she would predict that the patient would die, if it was absent then she predicted that he would live. Her observations were witnessed by leading men within the community to verify what she had seen.

"After the pig had been cooked a part of the intestine would be put in the hole with the blood and this would be covered with the black stone. This action was intended to keep the malevolent ghost who was causing the sickness in the hole.

"The power of this female ritual expert came from the Payame Ima and was passed down from mother to daughter over the generations."

b. Au with a Cure for Witchcraft (Sept. 18, 1991)

"*Kiapo kiano*—rubbing the *kiapo* ground on a person's body who is sick can reveal objects such as bamboo, flint, or red *hare* earth. These objects can be the signs that a witch has put these things inside of the person. An expert named Sisa could be gone to for help on this kind of illness. Sisa would say that he wanted to sleep, but really he wanted to dream and see what he could see. He would wake and say, 'I will hold the *ndele rowa* [divination stick].' He would be led by the *ndele rowa* to the house of a woman who had already had a child or several children but not to a woman who had no children. He would ask that a straight *soro* tree stick be brought to him, saying, 'You must not go the place of a *tama* (spirit) to cut the stick. If you do then it will interfere with the use of the stick. Bring the stick and make a fire. Bring pig grease. Hold the stick at one end and put the other end into the pig grease.' The spirits of the dead ancestors came onto the stick and would help in the hunt for the witch. The expert

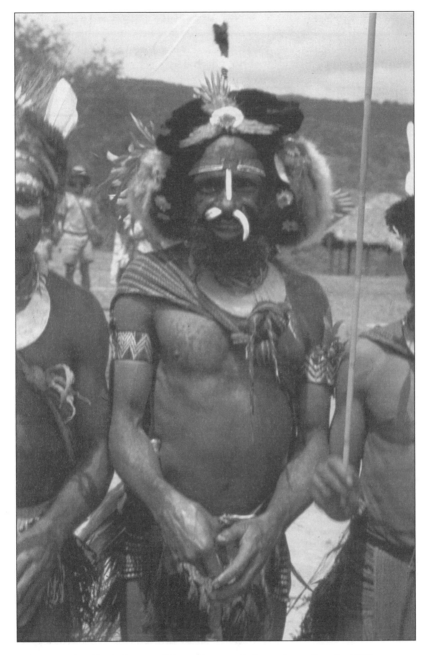

Figure 5–3. Au-Huri, decorated for a dance at Independence Day in 1991.

would say to the ancestors, 'Come and eat the pig grease and sit on this stick.' Sisa would then hold the *ndele rowa* and he would find a *pepe rowa* (another kind of stick) that a witch had stuck into the ground. The *pepe rowa* was a protection against the witch being discovered, a form of *kwei* (magical substance). She was going to kill the man and wanted to do so undiscovered. The expert would remove the witch's stick and plant another type of *kwei* stick onto which he would affix a woman's skirt [to block her witchcraft].

The expert would hold out the *ndele rowa* and it would find a woman who had several children. The *ndele rowa* would be held straight out from the expert and it would point at the finger of the accused woman and the expert would say, 'that is the finger that planted the *kwei*.' While he was holding this *ndele rowa* he asked the woman if she had planted the stick that he found and if she made the man sick. Then he told her not to look at the man again...He would tell witches not to look at men and eat them but eat pork instead.

After that pigs would be killed and a *tawanda* ritual would be performed for the sick man. Plenty of men and women would come for this but the accused witch would be told to sit by herself and not with others. Long strips of meat would be cut and offered to her and she would be told, 'Eat this and not the man.' Sometimes an accused witch would be isolated in the heat of the sun and under public gaze to prevent her from using her witchcraft. The relatives of the sick person would go to give a bundle of vegetable greens to the witch [and get her to withdraw her malevolent, consuming power].

Commentary: The description shows us that male and female experts were both involved in handling sickness and there was a cooperative division of labor between them. The ritual paraphernalia they used were fairly standard: types of earth (yellow, white clay), leaves (wild, cultivated, boundary markers like cordylines), and water (a fundamental element in fertility). Their actions aimed to determine what had *intruded* into the body and then after removing the objects to determine by *divination* what personalistic agency/agencies had caused sickness and whether death would result. Sacrificial offerings to dead kin aimed to recover the spirit of the sick person. The Payame Ima was a figure of cosmic proportions, associated with high forests, lakes, lightning, and rain, who also gave healing and divinatory powers to humans. As Au's second text shows, after the curer had removed objects from a sick person's body, another expert took over and sought out the witch in order to get her/him to withdraw the witchcraft and enable the patient to recover.

3. Sorcery and Healing

a. Pake on Kaliatauwi (Sept. 28, 1991)

"*Kaliatauwi* [the treatment for a condition in which the patient's legs were disjointed and he could not walk properly] involved killing pigs and the taking of pig grease and hiding in the forest in a cave away from all the walking paths in the area. Sugar cane, cordyline, taro corms and wood for lighting a fire would be brought to the cave. Two men would light a fire and put pig grease into the fire. The lengths of sugar cane that had been brought in would be broken into two and hung at either side of the patient. The expert would recite spells called *auwi* in which he named fruit pandanus, *angu* (sugar cane), and the *suku* banana. These were the names of foods that were not to be shared with anyone else after this ritual performance had been completed—this was a taboo. Also, the backbone/tail of the pig could not be shared with others.

"For four months the patient could not see people but had to stay away from them in the isolated place of the ritual. He would make a bush house in the area and stay there for some time and then later go out from the place. He was told not to look at women with children during this time [females who have given birth to children are potential witches]. The patient was told not to share sugar cane or banana with anyone unless they also had been through this ritual. After having gone through the ritual, a person could recount this curing spell while placing a stone on an enemy's footprint and cause them to have an injured limb or to be killed.

"Women who suffered from broken bones or wounded joints could also undergo this ritual but they were taken into the isolated bush area along with their husbands. Not many women did this. It was mostly a ritual for men. The name Kaliatauwi is specific to our area here. The neighbouring areas have different names for similar rituals. This ritual knowledge could be bought from knowledgeable persons. It was not simply passed down from father to son."

b. Pake on Mandi Auwi (Oct. 2, 1991)

"Two men were the teachers in this. They would find a red leaf and a white leaf and fasten these onto a stick. Then they would kill a pig and cut the backbone/tail out and remove the kidneys. These things would be taken to the cult site—a place where no pathways went in the deep bush. There they would make a house with two rooms and they would put the pig in the middle of this house. They would cook the pig. The men who were to be initiated into the *Mandi Auwi* would not eat the meat but would wait. The meat would be cut and wrapped with leaves along with grease into packets. The packets would be set aside in one of the rooms. *Mandi* is the name of the stick that was used in this ritual. The men inside would now invite the initiates into the house and they would beat them as they entered, hitting them with the *mandi* stick. Then the men would give the pork to them when they were all inside. The hitting of the initiates was accompanied by magical spell recitations—*sipu, sipu* [meaning unclear]. The stick that was used for the beating was hidden until the initiates had eaten their pork, then it was brought out and shown to the boys with more magical talk—*kika, kika, kika* ('hand holding'). At this point all the boys exited the house together.

The purpose of this ritual was so that the blood of these boys would stay young and would not become dry; so that they would not be sick but stay healthy. This ritual was conducted before the boys married. At this time the boys would shift from living solely in the women's house with their mother to living in the men's house, although they could still visit both houses at this time. This was like a school for young boys. It changed their blood and renewed it. If a boy did not go through this ritual he would not grow.

Commentary: The *Kaliatauwi* and *Mandi Auwi* narratives from Pake stand in nice counterpoint to each other. Both take the form of initiation rites. In the first it is a sick person who is secluded. The items brought to bear on the patient all have strong *joints*, especially the sugar cane. The long period of seclusion would in fact allow the bones to heal. In *Mandi Auwi* it was the growth of boys that was sought, again through seclusion, with both feeding and beating to stimulate and renew the blood. That healing rites for sickness and growth rites for boys should show the same ritual form is consonant with the fact that rituals for sickness belonged to a cosmic structure of reproduction among the Duna (compare Telban 1997).

c. Pake on Curing Ritual (July 19, 1991)

"When a man was sick and close to dying an expert would use magic to cure him. Four taro corms would be cooked in a fire. The taro would then be broken into eight or ten pieces. Two men would sit down on either side of the sick man who would be surrounded by the pieces of cooked taro. The man who had cooked the taro would step over *(takiya)* the sick man. Then a pig would be killed. They took part of the pig's heart and roasted it in ashes and they would preserve some of the pig's blood for later use.

"The sick man would sit down in the middle of these men. The taro that had been cooked had not yet been scraped of its outer skin. The expert would take a cassowary bone and scrape the taro while making a spell:

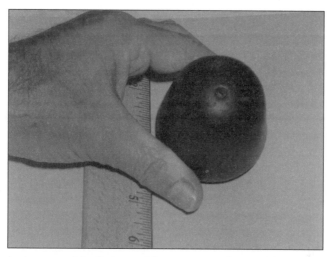

Figure 5–4. A stone, *tsiri ndewa*, used for curing ritual among the Duna.

Papumi and Lupumi,
Petame and Peyame....
Where will you go?
Blood flows from the nose into the hole.
Where will you go?
The Parotia birds all cry out,
The birds all cry out,
The birds all cry out,
The Honeyeater birds all cry out.
Down, down, down, down.
The wild nut pandanus tree is firmly rooted,
Strong rocks are firmly placed,
Wild pandanus is rooted,
Wild pandanus is rooted.
Strong rocks stay ,
Wild pandanus is rooted.
Down, down,down, down.
All the birds together cry out,
All the birds cry out:
Down, down,
'Go down there and arrive!
Go and arrive at your house-grove,
Go and come up to your pig stalls,
At the stalls of your pigs,
At the place where the *kitala* fruit pandanus grows,

> Go into your house-grove, under the eaves of your house,
> Come, and arrive!
> When you come, I will give you
> Something.*'

[* I.e., taro or pork, offered to the sick person on the tip of a cassowary bone. The spell begins with an appeal to the Payame Ima spirits to let the sick person's spirit return home from the land of the dead. The spell addresses the spirit, inviting it to come back and rejoin its owner's body. A version of this text appears also in A. Strathern 1996.]

"The ritual expert would recite this spell and take a part of the pork and taro and touch them to his armpit. He would take a seedling of pandanus and plant it calling to the *tini* (spirit) of the sick person to come back. Then a torch would be extinguished by thrusting it into the earth.

"Some of the pig's blood had been retained because a sorcerer or witch could have harmed the sick person by drying up their blood and the pig's blood could be used to replenish the sick person's blood.

"The spell called on the names of trees and birds and mountain crags where spirits of sick people have been driven. The spell asked that the *tini* be directed back to the sick person so that they could recover. In the spell the expert first calls on Papumi and Lupumi, two Payame Ima (Female Spirits) who live in the forested areas. These Female Spirits are called when spells are made because this magic originated with them. These Payame Ima go and sit with the *tini* of the dead. They are the keepers of the dead. The spell aims to get the Payame Ima to help in sending the sick person's *tini* back. The spell calls on nut pandanus and birds. These birds also cry out in order to send the spirit back to the living. [The evocative elements in this spell are similar to those in lament songs that women sing after the death of a community member (Stewart and Strathern n.d.).] As the *tini* of the sick person comes back from the high mountain area, home of the Payame Ima, that it has gone to the spell follows its progress on the journey from the mountain to domesticated gardens near the community houses.

"The pandanus tree is planted because it has roots which are strong and last a long time. Thus, the life of the patient should be firmly rooted and last a long time. That is why the nut pandanus is called in the spell.

"A fence is constructed after the *tini* has returned and the *tini* is told to stay inside and not to fly away again. The cane torch that had been extinguished in the ground was to frighten away the *tama* (spirit) that was making the person sick. The *tama* would be afraid of the light and go away. Also, the ritual expert would have red and black paint on his face while conducting the ritual which would make him look like a *tama* and perhaps also frighten away the *tama* that was causing sickness.

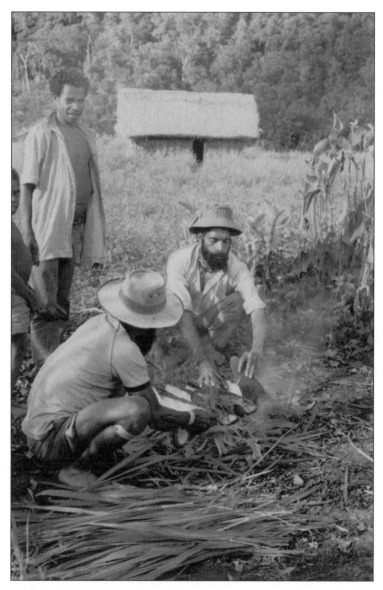

Figure 5–5. (1991) Kiliya—Hipuya prepares pandanus fruits for cooking. Kiliya is an expert on the esoteric aspects of knowledge, including witchcraft.

It was men who conducted this ritual of calling back the *tini*."

Commentary: Bodily sickness could often be the result of spirit loss. The spirit might travel to the land of the Payame Ima spirits in the high forest and had to be called back from there. The whole landscape is involved in this altitudinal vision of healing and the return of the spirit to the body. The sense of the cosmos is again vividly conveyed.

d. Urane on Traditional Medicine (March 29, 1991)

In the old days before white men came to the area people believed in the use of water, stones, and the killing of pigs to stop illness. Ritual experts would go and look at the sick man and ask him what part of the body was causing the trouble. The patient would say if it was the rib cage or chest, etc. The expert wanted to help the patient with the aid of magic—our people believed in this magic before. When a person was sick they invited experts in to help. The name of this was *ita kuma* ('pig nose') or *tama samu* (spirit spear) which referred to rib-cage pain or fever. This would arise when the spear of the spirit struck the sick person [i.e. in this part of the body]. The expert would work magic, *kao*. Some women knew of this magic but generally men knew it. There would be a pig killed and the expert would be happy and he would use medicine from the area that he was from to cure the sick person. He would use taro leaves and things like that, mixed with earth and rubbed on the areas that were painful. If a stone or bamboo knife was found to come out of the body from the rubbing it was a woman [i.e. a witch] that had put it there. These objects would have caused the pain that the patient experienced and thus they were removed. The father and friends of the expert would pay for this service and the expert would leave. This ritual knowledge would be passed down from father to son over the generations or from mother to daughter through teaching.

Menstrual blood could also make a man sick. In the past there were ways to cure this type of poisoning. Nowadays there is no way to treat this complaint.

Commentary: Urane's knowledge of traditional medicines was greatly reduced by comparison with that of Au and Pake who are senior knowledgeable male leaders. He is from a village near to the government station in Kopiago and is an Aid Post Orderly. He spoke in Tok Pisin rather than Duna and clearly distanced himself from the topic, aligning himself 'on the European side' in accordance with his training. His testimony shows respect for the traditional culture at the same time as demonstrating how attenuated knowledge of it is today. People come to the Aid Post not only because they accept biomedicine but also because they lack the older forms of knowledge of how to deal with sickness. The older men's knowledge is not being passed on to the newer generation of adults.

e. Pake on Epidemic Sickness and Curing Before Contact With the Outside (July 3, 1991)

"There was a time when a big sickness came and many people died. Several people would die in one house and a funeral would be held and then others would die before the time of mourning was over. This sickness passed through villages from the Lake Kopiago area. A wave of sickness passed from village to village. When it arrived here in Aluni people in Horaile [a neighboring parish] were already dying. We collected the skulls of dead dogs [dogs guard against witchcraft attacks] and painted them with red paint [a symbol of health in this culture] and erected them at the border between our village and Horaile at the place Yendei, in an attempt to stop the spread of the sickness.

"Then the people returned to the village and made a *sole tse* (curing dance). Three or four men would hold hands and dance in a circle with women behind them. But people still got sick with headache or coughing. This *kene kene* (death, death) epidemic still entered into our community. People also had *kene kene saiya* and malaria - *ipunaki*. These sicknesses came quickly and attacked people. Often a number of people in one household would die.

"I remember this type of sickness coming three times into the area when I was young. This would come from the Koroba direction beyond the nearby villages — from the south-east [where the Australians had set up administrative centers earlier]. Pigs were sick also and had yellow grease in their flesh [perhaps a sign of anthrax which was also known to have moved through the neighboring Enga region]. Pigs would just die. Another name for this is *towaleka*.

"As people died pigs were killed as sacrifices, and *kamo kamo* spells were recited. A sharp cassowary bone knife would be used to cut up the heart of the sacrificed pig and this would be fed to the sick person. This was called *tika*. Only married men could eat this pig's heart. Magical spells were also spoken at this time and a particular leaf would be rubbed on the chest of the sick person. The leaf was used by a ritual expert to divine if the person was going to die or live. The expert could actually determine when the sick person would die if he was not going to recover, such as early morning or sundown."

Commentary: Epidemics of sickness affecting both people and pigs swept across the Highlands of Papua New Guinea from east to west accompanying the early exploratory movements of prospectors and the extension of administrative control from the 1940s onwards (see Meggitt 1973: 111–113). The wave reached the Duna late, perhaps in the 1950s, before administrative control was established in the 1960s. It is interesting that in one narrative, by the male leader Male-Kaloma, it is said that the people attributed the epidemic to the same set of *tama* spirits they had placated before; while Pake mentioned that they had thought two new *tama* brought the *kene kene* sicknesses, called Yelipana and Kelipana. Given that the directional flow of epidemics was east to west and that outbreaks of human and porcine anthrax, pneumonia, and dysentery had occurred throughout the Enga area east of Duna in the 1940s, it is interesting to note the names of two spirits in an account from the Paiela (Ipili) area just to the east of the Duna-speaking territory. The two Paiela spirits are Elapi and Kelapi "who keep the earth and sky joined at the horizon" (Meggitt 1957:54). The Ipili thought these two spirits were rewarded "by unknown natives" (ibid.) with a feast of pigs and the sacrifice of a newborn child, otherwise their spells to uphold the cosmos would cease. Benevolent-spirits-turned-malevolent as a result of the lack of human offerings might well be imaged as the bringers of a disastrous epidemic from the horizons of the known world. The names of the two spirits are also reminiscent of those for two high mountains far to the east of the Duna in the Hagen area, also invoked in spells there as Kili and Yali (Giluwe and Ialibu).

4. Events of Witchcraft in 1998

The following narrative was provided to us by a married couple, Mr. Joseph-Tukaria and Mrs. Kesina-Kendoli. Upon our arrival into the field area in July 1998 we were greeted by Kesina's laments of mourning for two of their children. Duna women specialize in a form of cry songs which aim at sending the *tini*, spirit, of the deceased on to the places that dead spirits inhabit rather than remaining among the living where they can potentially cause sickness and, as is clearly evident in our translations of Kesina's songs (P.J. Stewart and A. Strathern n.d), remain too close to the grieving emotions of the living to allow recovery of the mourners' sense of well-being.

As soon as we entered our field house we were told that 'trouble' had come up in 1998 and that we needed to hear the story from them as soon as possible. The next day we were told the following:

"In 1997 a great time of hunger came up and in April of this year [1998] a 'trouble' came up. We had four children, Leti, Liniti, Joti, and Fredi. The

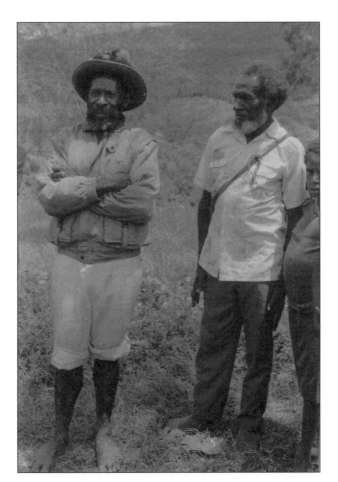

Figure 5–6. (1991) Pake-Kombara (at left) and Pastor Tukaria, Joseph's father.

last child was a boy whom we named Fredi. On the fourth day of the fourth month many people got very sick and we didn't have a doctor. The doctor [this reference is to the Aid Post Orderly not an actual doctor] was sick in Mendi [a city far away from the Aluni Valley, more than a day's car journey from Lake Kopiago] and didn't come back.

"None of us had any way to obtain medicine. Some of the sick people were taken to Kopiago but others who had no kin there stayed back in their own villages. We wanted to go to Kopiago but Kesina was close to dying and Tukaria [Joseph's father] was nearly dead too. Ben [one of Joseph's brothers] was sick and close to death as was Kesina's mother, our 'adopted' son, Olo and all of our children. I [Joseph] was also sick but sporadically only.

We decided we had to go to Kopiago station (a day's walk away) to seek medical assistance. I carried Fredi and a youth, Yeiye, carried Joti. We were all so sick we went very slowly on the journey. We stopped at Horaile [half way to Kopiago] and slept there overnight. The next morning we sent several people ahead to Kopiago to see if the Health Centre Car [a vehicle functioning as a local ambulance] could come and pick up my family from Horaile. The advance party was told that the bridge was out at the Tumbudu river and vehicles would not be able to cross over to Horaile. In addition the Health Centre car was not available anyway since it was in Mendi and not in Kopiago. So we had to travel on foot. We were able to use a canoe which provided a short cut for us across the lake and then we arrived at the *haus sik* [health center]. But the Aid Post Orderlies were not working, they were playing billiards. I said, 'my children are close to death, will you help me?' The reply was that they would help shortly. Urane [an Aid Post Orderly who had previously worked at Aluni, the village across from Joseph's village] came and asked a nurse to help us but the nurse didn't do much and just told us to wait in the *haus sik*.

"My little girl, Joti was very close to dying. She needed to defecate but was too weak to walk so I carried her out of the *haus sik*. Her neck at this time was bent way back [in a pose that Joseph later told us was an unnatural one and indicated that witches were pulling her head backwards to cut her throat]. I carried her back into the *haus sik* where she expired. This was day eight [four days after the sickness was reported to have arisen]. At this time the Health Centre car returned and took us to a house where Kesina's brother, Keni, lives in the village of Hirane. We all began mourning the death of Joti even though we ourselves were still very sick. Two days later we returned to Hagu and buried Joti.

"The day after the burial I said that I would kill a pig and steam-cook it and I said, 'If there is a woman with witchcraft here you cannot kill our boy Fredi.' Kesina and I both said, 'We don't want to mourn another child. We don't know if witchcraft killed Joti or not but we don't want this boy to die.' We spoke out publicly. During that night Fredi was very sick. In the morning we cooked the pig and divided the pork out to be eaten [Joseph was offering the witches whom he suspected of killing and eating Joti pork to eat instead of the boy Fredi]. I said, 'You women must each hold this child and pray, you must eat this pork and sleep in this house—no one must go from this house' [this was aimed at keeping the witches from using their powers to kill the boy]. After this talk I fell asleep. I had been so busy up to this point that I had not slept for four or five days. When I awoke almost everyone had gone away. Fredi was cold and I took him out into the warm air and sat with him. Tears came into his eyes and he clung onto my shoulder. Then his head bent backwards and he died [here again Joseph later told us that the head of the child being bent backwards was a sign that the child was killed by witches].

"We mourned and all of the relatives came back after they heard that the boy too had died. I asked my father if Fredi should be buried at Kopiago [where the boy's mother's kin are from] but he said that he himself was old and would be dying soon and said, 'Let this one stay near his sister.'

"Shortly after Fredi's death an angry relative came saying, 'I want to kill one of these witches and bury her like Fredi.' This man pulled out a bush knife as though to kill several of the women who were suspected of having killed Joti and Fredi but we restrained him saying, 'Don't—we'll ask these women if their witchcraft truly killed these two children or not. We will ask them, so you must not kill them.' We assigned one man to go and ask the suspected women but he was afraid to do so, but two other men were not afraid and did go to do this [one of these men had lost a small child during the epidemic and thought that witchcraft had killed the child].

"One woman who was questioned said that yes, she and several others had killed these children. This woman spoke out—confessed—and she named the other four female witches who were also involved in killing and eating the children. She was asked why these witches wanted to kill Joti and Fredi and she gave three reasons: (1) That Joseph [who is the sole representative of the agnatic *anoagaro* line and therefore in a particularly powerful situation in relation to issues of land use] would not let a garden be planted on a particular plot of land that had bush growing on it saying that the land belonged to someone else and it could not therefore be used by others for gardens. (2) That Kesina has a sewing machine and makes nice dresses which she wears and sells for money and that they were jealous of this. (3) That Joseph's family wore new clothes and that worried them (i.e., they were jealous).

"Alright, I said, 'she spoke out and named those involved, if you ask any more questions there will be more trouble so this is enough. The boy will be buried first and then I will publicly make a speech about this confession and what will be done. Tomorrow we would normally prepare an earth oven cooking of pandanus and pumpkin [two foods that are abundant in the area and frequently eaten] but now I have to take Kesina to the *haus sik*.' Kesina was confused and very sick and told the people to go away. I said, 'The two children will have to stay here— the dead ones —Joti and Fredi will have to stay here. We will go. Five women have been named as involved in these killings by witchcraft. Perhaps this is true or perhaps not—we will find this out and in the last days God will reveal the truth. If in the future I no longer live here I want the bush to cover this place over. I don't want any of you to live here because I don't know if my boy was killed by witchcraft or not [Joseph again is referring to his special status in the community in relation to land use].'

"I was asked by Dokoya, a senior man, if I was saying that these suspected witches must go back to their places or if these women must leave and take their husbands with them. I said, 'The women with witchcraft must go. If you women don't have witchcraft then don't go. As for you men, you do not have to go. It was these women who sinned and I'm not happy about this.'

"During the time that this was going on the son of one of the accused witches suddenly came and struck his mother, kicking her in the chest. The woman died from this blow and was taken to her house and buried. We did not call the witches' names. It had been one of the witches herself who called these other women's names. The man killed his mother himself.

"At this time all of those who had come to mourn the death of Fredi ran away with the exception of two or three people such as Keni. A meeting was called at the communal men's house. I said that the son had killed his mother in an unprovoked manner and that we were not responsible for this because 'the man himself did this deed.' But it was decided that I and Kesina's brother must pay compensation payments to the kin of the woman who had been killed by her son. The verdict was that four times fourteen items (probably pigs) plus 200 kina cash must be paid by us to the kin of the dead woman. The man who murdered his mother was told to pay four times fourteen items and 200 kina cash to this family and that he would not be put in jail if these compensation payments were made. It was also decided that the kin of the murdered woman would kill two or three pigs for the two dead children, Joti and Fredi, because the witch's son himself killed his mother without any guidance from his own kin and this forced us (Joseph and Kesina's family) to pay a large compensation to the suspected witch's family. This was very difficult because the Christians don't want to help [the church condemns the practice of involvement in compensation payments arising from witchcraft cases]. Some people did help us though. If they had not helped I would have just worried about this. Even though the four times fourteen items have been paid the cash amount of 200 kina is still owing.

"I had thought that Joti was going to die. She grew very quickly and was large and healthy. Also, the boy Fredi was really fat and all the men in the community were very devoted to him [these images of the children being fat and large are ones meant to imply that they were attractive to witches who like to eat human flesh].

"It was not just our children who died this year. Plenty of children between the ages of six months and three years of age died at approximately this same time. In addition some old people died, two old women and one old man. This sickness that came is called *kenekene* (death death) [this is the same name that was given to the epidemic sicknesses that preceded the first whites coming into the area]. The symptoms included shortness of breath, sleepiness, general body weakness, and fever.

"Although plenty of people died we were concerned about witchcraft having killed Joti and Fredi for two reasons: (1) Two siblings dying in one week is not usual. (2) Both the children had their necks pulled backwards in the fashion that witches turn a victim's neck prior to killing them. Also, last week I sought the advice of a *kerane anoa* (prophet). This prophet is a Bimin [i.e. from across the Strickland river beyond Duna territory] man who had previously come to the community to help determine what had happened in the case of a boy who had gone missing. This prophet had come and determined that some witches had killed this boy and put his body remains in a river, placing a large stone on top of his body so that it would not float up and be found. This prophet man has the ability to determine these things and can speak out publicly.

"First the *kerane anoa* and I prayed. Then he asked me how the children had died and if the neck was bent backwards at death. Kesina and I didn't ask him about this. He asked it himself and when we said that yes the neck had been bent backwards he said that it was witches who had done this. We called out the names one by one of these witches and asked if they had witchcraft and he confirmed that these women did have witchcraft. He told us that these witches had eaten the children and he showed us how the witches had cut the bodies up and eaten them. We believed this prophet and we paid him 10 kina for his help. [This category of ritual expert here called a prophet existed in the past and was given the powers to determine who were witches by the use of a stick called the *ndele rowa*. These powers were said to have been given to special men by the Female Spirit, *Payame Ima*.]

At this point Kesina added this part of the story:

My head was not working well. People in the community came and complained to us about this trouble that had come up and the accusations about witchcraft so I got up to show them that they had no reason to be jealous of us anymore. I broke everything—the sewing machine, saucepans and dishes. I burnt the mattress and blankets—everything. These people were jealous of us so I destroyed these things and now we do without them [the witches were said to have killed the two children, Joti and Fredi, because they were jealous of the belongings of Joseph and Kesina]. I said to them, 'If you're complaining about these things you can have them all and go about your business without harming us' [Kesina had told us that she was worried that her remaining two children would also be killed and eaten by jealous witches]. We covered everything in kerosine and burnt it. We put the remnants of the destroyed objects under the house here so that everyone could see that these objects were ruined and of no use to us. We want to leave all this trouble behind us.

Commentary: This remarkable and poignant case history shows clearly the confused interplay of pluralistic ideas and practices today, involving attributions of witchcraft, attempts to use biomedical resources, and ecological stress. It stands in fitting counterpoint to the narratives of precolonial epidemics and attempts to cope with them, and indicates how old practices return in new guises with conflations of indigenous and Christian ideas: the essence of both pluralism and conflict.

*   *   *

Pluralism has appeared frequently in the ethnographic accounts so far. In the next chapter we consider it directly as a phenomenon, using data from the Huli area which lies to the south of where the Duna live.

Chapter 6

Medical Pluralism

Biomedical medicine and indigenous systems of medicine are often assumed to be in conflict with one another. Indigenous practices may be seen as blocking or interfering with the progress of modern medical treatment regimes. But various contexts exist in which introduced and indigenous medical practices meet different requirements for the population in question. In this instance, then, the two systems are seen to be complementary rather than in conflict. Also, introduced medicine may not be wholly or in some instances even partially beneficial in the final analysis. In all areas of the world, however, as globalization makes shared forms of knowledge more widely available, some aspects of western medicine may be accepted, while others are rejected.

Medical pluralism exists in any arena where competing forms or systems of medical practices coexist. Individuals therefore make decisions when selecting a particular form of medical treatment. These decisions may be influenced by a consideration of the treatment offered, the relative costs involved, or the religious and political environment in which the person lives. Although there is a universal basis of experience as a biological phenomenon, the perceived causes, treatments, and consequences of injury or illness are greatly affected by culture.

Stephen Frankel (1986) has described how the Huli people of the Southern Highlands of Papua New Guinea view illness. Frankel brings a unique perspective to his anthropological investigation of Huli ideas about illness since he trained as a biomedical doctor prior to conducting his ethnographic work.

The Huli

The Huli people were first contacted by whites in the 1930s and efforts were made by the Australian Administration in the 1950s to control warfaring between the various Huli groups. These people are a large, agriculturally based population who rear pigs and intensively cultivate sweet potato. They have had to some extent and still do have elaborate ideas about the decline of the earth and its fertility and the need to renew the

93

earth's fertility at regular intervals (approximately every thirteen generations) by a ritual called the *dindi gamu* cycle. The cyclicity of this ritual may
be attached to the oral history of volcanic ash falls in the past (Frankel
1986: 16–17; Ballard 1994). This ash fall is predicted to occur again at a
time when the earth will be run down and there will be a profusion of epidemic diseases. According to the ritual lore, the Huli saw themselves as
descended from an ancestor, Hela, who also fathered other groups of people in the wider area. The Huli borrowed rituals and customs from these
neighbors who were related through descent from Hela. *Dindi gamu* lore
tells of a flow of ritual power across the landscape of the Hela peoples
that is joined by a root system that passes through underground streams
(Frankel 1986: 16–26). This sort of ritual trackway is also found in other
areas of Papua New Guinea (P. Stewart 1998).

The Huli have also been extensively missionized by Catholic and other
Churches, which has had profound effects on religious practices and ideas.
Some three to ten generations ago, a boy, Bayebaye, is said to have been
killed in error at a ritual occasion and as his mother left the area and went
north to Duna she cursed future generations. Bayebaye is likened nowadays to Christ. The name means "perfect" and refers to a harmonious cosmological state in which there is fertility of crops, pigs grow well, and
people are healthy — a state the Huli aspire to recover (Frankel 1986:
23–26).

At the time of contact when whites entered into their territory, the Huli
suffered terribly from epidemic diseases which disrupted social, political,
and religious structures. These epidemics were attributed to the arrival of
new *dama* spirits (i.e., the white people). Nowadays, the Huli say that
they are more subject to bronchitis, anthrax, venereal diseases, and malaria
(*wabi warago*). The exposure to all of these diseases is thought by epidemiologists to have first occurred, or to have increased, when explorers
of European descent first came into the area. The increase in malaria is
perhaps to be correlated with the movement of mosquitoes and their eggs
along with the gear of these whites.

In 1960–61, the Huli began to be exposed more to patrols by Australian
administrators who were given the task of "pacifying" the local people
and bringing them under administrative control. At this time Huli people
were experiencing a high degree of anxiety over the rapid and often confusing changes in their society that accompanied the entry of the whites
into the area. A period of "madness" (*lulu*) occurred in which people be-
haved in unpredictable ways and experienced dizziness and confusion. A
similar type of madness occurred in another Highlands area, Pangia, at
approximately the same time and was brought on by a parallel set of con-
founding circumstances in which the people found themselves unable to cope
(A. Strathern 1977; P. Stewart and A. Strathern 1997a).

"Saints, Cargocar and Cchiz... mental illness and stress"

At a later time, the Huli began a museum/cultural center, whose real purpose was to restore *dindi gamu*, in part because they were disturbed by changes in adolescents' growth patterns in which they observed that they were maturing at an earlier age. This overearly maturation was taken to be a sign that an imbalance existed in the cosmological scheme and needed to be redressed through the enactment of the *dindi gamu*. This attempt at reviving the ritual was supported by many local people, but the impact of Christianity on the Huli has altered their ways of establishing a cosmological balance. The indigenous notion of harmful spirits, *dama*, was incorporated into the teaching of the missionaries who used the term interchangeably with "Satan." The notion of the periodic decline of the earth and its people has also been incorporated into Christian ideology. Thus, the Last Days are expected from time to time. There was a period of concern with this early in 1976, and there was much glossolalia, healing, and confession of sin. The 1983 eclipse of the sun brought similar responses. The complex mixture of indigenous and introduced beliefs has impacted all arenas of Huli life including their ideas of disease and health in general.

The Huli conception of health is a state of resistance to illness or disease which might intrude into their lives. They see health as a condition that must be striven for through the use of ritual knowledge and prudent living. Illness results from one's lack of caution or from another's wrongdoing. In particular (like other Highland peoples of Papua New Guinea) they are concerned with health as a means of attracting wealth and influence. Lengthy training in the bachelor's cult (*ibagiya*) was directed towards this end and designed to strengthen young men for adult life and marriage. These cults were organized by adult bachelors who were specialists in this job. The cult aimed at making the young boys handsome and providing them with a good skin through the use of spells and herbs. These were thought to be able to give strength and power to the youths so as to increase their success as warriors (Frankel 1986: 97–123). Here as in many parts of Papua New Guinea a good skin is visually attractive and symbolizes the moral qualities inside the person. There is no clear separation between the physical appearance and the moral state of the individual. Socially marginalized persons tend to be identified with those who are unhealthy. These sorts of bachelor cults were also performed in the neighboring Duna area where boys were secluded in growth houses (*palena anda*) (P. Stewart and A. Strathern 1997b).

For the Huli dying is a fluid state; and mourning can begin before the person is dead. When people are ill, they often simply say *homedo* (I am dying). *Homaya*, he died, is a term that can be used to refer to a corpse or to someone who had been extremely ill but who has subsequently recovered (Frankel 1986: 59).

Frankel distinguishes several ways in which Huli act when sick: by doing nothing, attempting self-help, seeking Christian healing, or visiting aid posts (small facilities where an orderly works who has been trained to dispense some medicines, take temperatures, and perhaps give shots) and health centers (facilities that provide more services than the aid post but fewer than a hospital). Frankel found that older men tended to do nothing when sick, more often than to seek some sort of treatment, while many other people used Christian healing. Mothers with children under five years of age took these children to aid posts quite frequently and children who were five to eleven years of age were very frequently taken as well. The health center in the area where Frankel was working was far away and therefore not used very often. Frankel gives a composite picture of choices people make in response to illness: symptoms ignored or treated at home, 64% of the cases; self-help, 4%; aid post, 24%; Health Center, 2%; and Christian healing, 6%. Frankel sees the Huli as rather pragmatic and the large number of cases where sickness was treated naturalistically as evidence of this. It may be noted, however, that where serious illness is involved, explanation becomes more important. And nowadays Christian pastors compete with the indigenous system through treatment of illness (pp. 75–80, 176). Western medicine can also usually be combined with other forms of treatment such as ritual or dispute settlement, and proof is sometimes sought for injury as a cause of sickness, thus bringing illness from private into public spheres by way of attributions of responsibility for conditions and the obligation or demand to pay compensation for them, perhaps many years after an injury is sustained.

Huli indigenous concepts of pain and blood are closely related. Blood is thought to be able to settle in a particular part of the body and cause pain. For example, chronic bronchitis may be ascribed to an old injury where blood had clotted and is thought to have ultimately produced phlegm. When a person is weak, he says that his blood is not doing its work, or that the blood inside him is finished. The same expressions are found among another Highlands Papua New Guinea people, the Melpa of Mount Hagen. A Huli person in pain may simply say *darama* (blood). A pain that moves through the body may be described as the flow of bad blood from one site to another. The Melpa similarly speak of blood pricking them by its movement (*mema poklpa morom*). Blood that bursts out of its proper place and settles at the base of the back can be said to cause pain, as can blood thought to enter into the belly to harden and clot there. These ideas are examples of humoral notions that a humor out of place causes imbalance, bad mixing, and sickness (see Ch. 3). There is another Huli expression that people use, saying that their blood has turned to water, and that this is a serious sign (pp. 82–83).

For the Huli, life, consciousness, intellectual activity, and moral sensibility result from the four principles which are important: *Bu* = breath or vital force. Because respiratory disease is dangerous, dyspnea is taken as a bad sign. *Mini* = thoughts, which derive from the *bu*. Those who lack a proper social consciousness are said to be without *mini*. *Manda* = memorized knowledge. *Dinini* = spirit, which detaches itself in sleep and in illness. These four components can be compared with the Melpa (Hagen) and Wiru (Pangia) people of the Highlands (see Table 1).

	Huli	Melpa	Wiru
Breath	Bu	Mukl-nga	Aru
Thoughts	*Mini*	Noman	Wene
Knowledge	Manda	Noman-nt pili	Wene toko
Spirit	Dinini	*Min*	*Yomini*

Table 1. Indigenous terms for four vital components of a person that affect wellness.

It can be seen from the table that in each culture there are terms that recognize the importance of all four elements to life and health. Breath is vital to life but in all cases is distinguished from spirit, also considered vital. Death occurs when spirit leaves the body and does not return (as in our folk term "giving up the ghost"). Thoughts and knowledge are closely connected: in Melpa understanding takes place in the *noman*, which can be translated as either "thoughts" or "mind" generally. In Wiru knowledge is "he or she makes thoughts." The term Frankel gives for knowledge in Huli, *manda*, may be eymologically related to Melpa *man* (advice, wisdom) and Wiru *mana* (sacred talk, the language of spells). In all three cultures bad thoughts can lead to sickness, which in turn can be corrected by knowledge. The morph *min* or *mini* appears in all three languages, but means "thoughts" in Huli, "spirit" in Melpa and Wiru.

In terms of environmental agents of disease, the Huli stress the action of worms (*ngoe*). Also, food fragments can stay in the stomach and cause illness. Malaria is described as the illness from the lowlands, doubtless accurately. Some sicknesses are said to be seasonal, e.g., colds. *Amali* is a stubborn cough (perhaps a sign of emphysema or tuberculosis) old men get that produces chronic chest pain, and they should not share tobacco pipes with others. All of these ideas can be paralleled among the Melpa, showing a commonality of experience and its interpretation cross-culturally in Highlands New Guinea.

Although traditional remedies are not used much nowadays by the Huli, there was in the recent past the use of sap, leaves, flowers, grass tips, and nettles in various curing practices. Scorched taro is still used for diarrhea (the charcoal is probably the useful active agent here).

For the Huli, as well as other Highlands societies in Papua New Guinea, illnesses can be grounded in social relations. For example, physical assaults that produce injuries can be at some later point in time linked with a sickness that arises in the previously injured person even though many years may have passed between the injury and the onset of the sickness. Frankel describes one case in which an old man was thrown to the ground and approximately one year later developed dysentery which he attributed to the prior incident by stating that the blood from that injury had moved down his body and was now producing the dysentery. In another case a woman attributed a headache that she had to a blow she had received twenty-five years earlier when her husband had hit her with a wooden plank. The person who makes such claims is seeking to obtain a payment (compensation) from the person or their kin who had previously injured them. In the above example the woman with the headache was given sixteen pigs by her husband's clan. The compensation payment thus serves as a cure for injury and subsequent illness that might arise from injury. This type of "curing" is found in various areas in Papua New Guinea and exists in a climate where interpersonal relationships routinely involve conflict and violence. Huli husbands are deterred from beating their wives sometimes by fear of having to pay compensation. Women sometimes threaten to commit suicide if treated too badly and in some instances actually do kill themselves. In one case a Huli woman left a sign that indicated her reasons for committing suicide and the husband's clan had to pay the dead woman's kin ninety pigs in compensation. In many of the violent disputes that arise between people, especially the domestic ones, the heightened emotional state of the injured participants may cause various illnesses (pp. 124–149).

Illnesses may be attributed to fright (*gi*), desire (*hame*), sorrow (*dara*), anger (*keba*), and spite (*madane*).

1. *Fright*. The word for startle implies that the spirit has left the body (*mogo lara*). This can cause illness, so anyone responsible for startling another may be blamed. This particularly holds in relation to young children, for whom the attachment of the spirit to the body is thought to be fragile. There is a similarity here with convulsions which some small children are susceptible to. Wives may accuse husbands of startling children and thus seek compensation, so the syndrome becomes part of a legal conflict between them.

2. *Desire*. If one person covets the food of another this may result in illness for the one whose food is desired. The hungry person swallows spittle (the same concept exists among the Melpa and Wiru) and the other falls sick. This form of desire that can lead to overconsumption is thought of in highly negative terms as representing uncontrolled greed, which is equated to the behavior of witches who attack humans because of their greedy nature.

Conditions of both fright and desire can be made worse by the presence of a *kuyanda* condition (a kind of tangled clot held to result from a child swallowing its mother's blood). *Hame* sickness, resulting from a covetous glance at food by another person is held, like fright, to occur mostly in children. There is a traditional treatment for it, but most Huli women are Christians nowadays, and thus do not use the cure for their children, preferring Western medicine.

3. *Sorrow.* Frankel tells an interesting story of an old man whose wife had just died. He had been very fond of her. "She stays in my lung" is the phrase for this. He was afraid she might come back and claim him because of his grief for her, and he was unable to sleep at night. Traditionally, he could have performed a ritual to protect himself, but he was now a Christian, and felt that he could not do so, and thus had to live with the fear. There is certainly stress felt by Huli widowers in general: they show an increased mortality rate in the first year of bereavement (p. 143).

4. *Anger.* Anger is involved in self-destructive behavior since anger may make the person who experiences it sick. Frankel explicitly makes the comparison with the Melpa here. However, for the Melpa there is a greater involvement of the ancestral spirits who may be seen as sending sickness to elicit sympathy for the one who is ill.

5. *Spite.* When let down by others, people feel *madane*, and they may make sorcery, which causes illness in the one they resent. The *dama* (spirit) Toro may be enlisted to help one make sorcery against those with whom one is angry. Toro is a spirit from the Duna area north of Huli. Other kinds of sorcery are said to come from the Duguba peoples to the south. There are practitioners to remove the effects of some types of sorcery. Nowadays people are increasingly afraid of sorcery from the coastal areas, *nambis poison*, especially feared by those who have returned from laboring work on the coast and have been in touch with men of other ethnic groups. In other cases, people do not specify who is making the sorcery against them, but in all cases it is assumed that anger or spite are involved.

In cases of attack by traditional *dama*, pork sacrifices were made to ensure recovery. Such sacrifices were also made to secure generalized fertility for people and crops. Datagaliwabe is a spirit who punishes transgressions between kinsmen. His qualities in turn dominate in the Huli conception of the Christian God. But God is supposed to punish for transgressions against non-kinsmen as well. And all *dama* are regarded as Satan, whereas traditionally some were nurturing as well. It is clear that sickness is now a contested terrain between religions. There is also an idea that if a traditional ritual is neglected for too long, the spirit becomes annoyed and may attack one with sickness, and this notion must increase the tension involved in the new struggle between indigenous and Christian ideas. Men may see particular spirits in dreams, which impels them to make certain sacrifices (pp. 144–149) so that dreams give an experiential drive to ritual activity and therapy.

Christians insist that people should not even talk of traditional religion, in case they become sick. God too is thought to be vengeful if neglected (very much an Old Testament view). Sometimes when people get better they ascribe this to their return to the church even though they have also had hospital treatment. Sacrifices to enlist the support of a spirit are largely replaced now by prayers, in line with the supposed conflict between God and all spirits as *dama*, incarnations of Satan.

Frankel illustrates the poignancy which the conflict of indigenous and introduced ideas brings with it. A widow fell ill with chest pain. She had not completed the mourning rituals for her dead husband, and so she felt his shade had attacked her. She had also made herself vulnerable to such an attack by marrying again. (In Hagen, a special pig is sacrificed in order to appease the spirit and take care of this problem, called the "pig of the widow's bridge.") She became seriously ill. She was treated in Tari Health Centre and recovered. The dead man's relatives also held a sacrifice and asked God to drive away his spirit. Frankel makes an observation which also applies elsewhere. "Another response for Christians to the quandary that strongly indicated ceremonies are forbidden to them is to allow others who are still 'heathens' to perform the ceremony for them" (p. 166).

Both indigenous and Christian teaching adhere to the belief that excessive emotion in itself is bad. One Huli woman that Frankel reports on was angry with her husband for not helping her with money. When her baby became sick, she thought God was punishing her for being angry. Christian women sometimes do not fight back physically, but if they get angry inside they will fall ill. This idea certainly sets a problem for them. Illness as coercion is a pattern found in the Huli material and in many other instances in the Highlands. Traditional moral ideas do endure as well in some ways. If a man commits adultery, his children's health is endangered. (This idea is also found in Pangia.) Such an idea may act to restrain people's behavior and hence support morality. From another viewpoint actual occurrences of sickness may lead to blame and coerced payments of compensation.

Effective presentation of self is important in Huli society, and health is required for this. It can be threatened by strong emotions which can cause illness. Hence people are wary about eliciting such feelings in others. And people are easily put at risk, also "society [is seen] as under constant threat from the disorder that may follow the conflicting wishes of its members" (p. 185). Frankel also notes a continuity and interweaving of ideas which modifies the applicability of the concept of pluralism to Huli practice. Nevertheless it is clear from the data that the Huli are in general in a highly pluralistic situation with regard to their medical choices.

Frankel takes the experience of illness to be a biological universal, although the management of this experience varies culturally. In particular cultures, conditions may be diagnosed that are not recognized in others (although they may perhaps be recognized as something else). He cites here the Huli category *kuyanda*, which is believed to result from a child swallowing its mother's blood. The blood is thought to settle in the chest as a parasitic mass and must be removed by a specialist. The ritual is likely to be done for a child born with blood in its mouth (Frankel, p. 101). Otherwise, Frankel is skeptical of examples given by writers of "culture-bound syndromes": conditions recognized as sicknesses by people but not recognizable as such in biomedicine. Frankel himself uses the standard distinction between disease as a biological entity and illness as a social process which we employ in this book, so he does recognize the disparity between these two concepts. He takes into account the common and newer conditions as well as the more serious illnesses, and this he does specifically so that his work may be useful in health planning for the area. He is also interested in exploring the Huli's response to introduced health care, as one would expect from someone trained both as a biomedical physician and an anthropologist.

Medical Pluralism in Hagen

For the Hagen (Melpa) people of Papua New Guinea, we see parallels with the Huli in evaluating the effectiveness of a new treatment before accepting it and in determining if a treatment fits into existing cultural logic. Throughout the history of contact in the Highlands, penicillin injections have been remarkably effective in getting rid of yaws, ulcers, and infections in wounds. As a result of this, the injection, or "shoot" is the most popular form of treatment requested by patients who visit aid posts, even in instances when it is not an appropriate form of treatment. A reverse example in Hagen is that a slim person is likely to be classified as "emaciated", "bone nothing," "without any body." Persons who are fat are seen to have enough money to eat more and thus through a conceptual tie between health and wealth to be healthy. For this resaon persons who are overweight and may be at risk of heart disease do not seek, or accept, medical advice on dieting.

Though injections have become accepted as a highly effective treatment for painful and life threatening diseases, the problem is that they are now assumed to be equally good for a range of other conditions, which may not require any sort of injection. The "shoot" has been classified as on a par with "magic" and therefore preferred over other sorts of treatment. Another reason for the popularity of injections is that they have no counterpoint in traditional medicine and are perceived as "strong" because they were introduced by the colonial powers who brought other "strong" things.

The idea that injections are the most powerful form of introduced medicine by no means implies that the whole western theory of what causes disease is either understood or accepted. Medical pluralism in the Highlands often results from two factors: (1) The acceptance of introduced practices without much understanding of the reasons for, or theory behind, them; and (2) the belief that there are certain conditions which are caused by entities outside of the worldview recognized by Western doctors and which, therefore, must be treated in a ritual way if the patient is to recover.

The first factor leads to people combining medical practices in an eclectic fashion with random results; the second to a positive choice to use traditional rather than introduced medicine in cases where the causes are held to be ones outside of Western purview. In addition, as an illness progresses and perhaps does not respond to one type of treatment, people are willing to switch to another type in the search for a cure. Traditional ritual, Christian prayers, and hospital treatment may all be involved in an all out effort to save a patient's life.

It is in the sphere of ritual that most questions arise regarding traditional medicine, some saying it is superstitious nonsense, others that it performs valuable therapeutic functions where there are psychosomatic aspects of illness. In such discussions it is important to explicate and differentiate the viewpoints of the participants from those of the observer or writer. The participants consider that medicine of any kind either works or it does not. In the case of Western medicine, it is thought to work because of the "strong power" of the people who invented it, in the case of their own medicine, it works because the spirit entities which cause illness are affected by the actions of ritual. Christian prayers, it is thought, may have an overriding effect on sickness because of the belief in the "miracle working power" of God. There is, however, a category of medicine in which belief is of much the same order whether it is Western or traditional remedies that are used, and that is plant medicines employed to counter minor body conditions such as skin rashes and boils or stomach pains and diarrhea. In all traditional medical systems there is a proportion of plants which do have beneficial effects of this kind, and it is commonplace to observe that important European synthetic medicines derive originally from plants used by rural peoples around the world. There were indeed numerous plants used in this way in the Highlands (A. Strathern 1989). Hageners have a strong theory, however, that sickness can be brought on directly by the state of a person's *noman* (mind). If a person experiences anger/frustration (*popokl*) in their *noman*, they may become sick. If a person becomes sick, people will ask if he or she has hidden some *popokl* and ask for it to be declared so that they can help to cure the person. If the sick person has been suffering from a sense of being wronged by others, the questioning provides an opportunity for the sick person to reveal grievances and perhaps have them removed by remedial action. The confession of these feelings can make the person feel better as well as reveal breaches of the Melpa moral code and help connect broken relations between people. From the point of view of the Hageners, for sickness to be cured, social relationships must first be properly sorted out.

This Hagen theory of *popokl* dovetails well with western theories of psychosomatic illness. The theory of *popokl* as a factor underlying the causes of illness does not interfere with the use of other forms of therapeutic treatment.

When a Hagener becomes ill, western biomedical treatments, Christian notions of healing, and indigenous religious concepts may all be applied. A benign combination of factors, however, does not always eventuate. One example is to be found in the sphere of "sorcery." If an illness is diagnosed as caused by a certain kind of sorcery involving soul-capture, it is held that no western medical treatment can possibly succeed against it. Such treatment may still be tried, but there is a fatalistic attitude towards it. Instead, much expense will be incurred in procuring ritual solutions.

The Wiru of Pangia

The best examples of this sorcery treatment process come from the Pangia area in the Southern Highlands Province, among the Wiru people. There are three types of sorcery recognized by the Wiru. One is *tomo*, which can almost be glossed as "poison." As it is thought to be ingested with food or drink, so it is appropriate that indigenous treatment should consist of a sacrifice plus the administering of a concoction to induce vomiting. Aid Post orderlies generally adhere to the local views, treat the category of *tomo* sickness as real, and apply emetics and laxatives as functional equivalents of the indigenous medicine. One orderly in fact believed for many years that his wife, a woman from an enemy clan to his own, regularly administered *tomo* and also love magic to him so that he would not look at other women. In counteraction, he made himself vomit. (Eventually, he married another wife and the first wife broke with him, much to his relief. His relatives commented on how much younger and healthier he looked thereafter.) *Tomo*, then, does not raise problems for health care, provided that it relates only to stomach upsets or other conditions which may be expected to correct themselves and not to be too adversely affected by making the patient vomit.

The second category of sorcery is called *nakenea*, and may be glossed as "leavings sorcery." Anything imbued with a part of the intended victim's substance can be used as the instrument of sickness here - a piece of clothing, chewed sugarcane, blood, fingernail, hair, excrement. The item must be picked up so that it does not touch the skin of the attacker, oth-

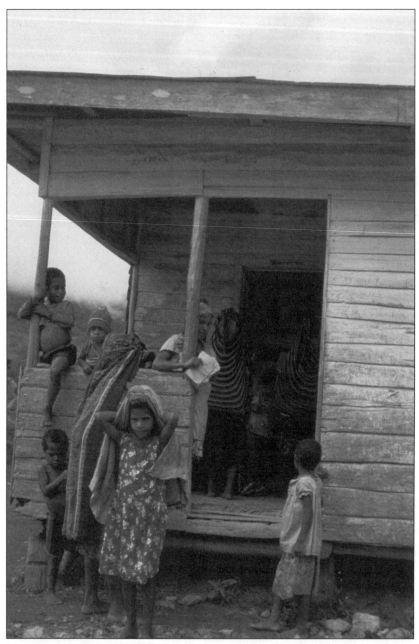

Figure 6–1. Women and children at the Aluni Aid Post, staffed in 1991 by Urane (Duna).

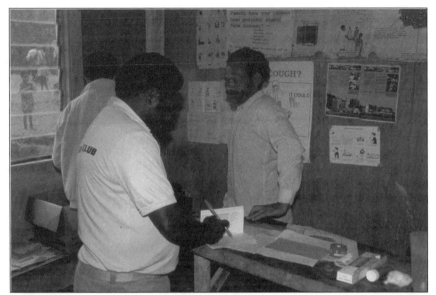

Figure 6–2. Inside the Aluni Aid post. Visiting orderlies are making family records (Duna).

erwise it would become imbued equally with the attacker's own substance. To prevent an item being taken for *nakenea* use in this way one would throw it into water: food remains are regularly disposed of in this way (a practice which might cause water pollution if carried out regularly). Once it has been taken the attacker wraps it with care and secretly transports it to a master sorcerer who hangs the package above a fire or a pool of water. As the fire burns up, so the victim sweats in fever, or, as the water rises, he shivers. The effects of *nakenea* can only be removed if the item is traced and recovered with expensive payments to the sorcerer. Effort is therefore definitely drawn away from hospital action as such.

The third kind of sorcery is held to be the most lethal and the most immune to western treatment. This is *sangguma*, or *maua/uro* in Wiru. The sorcerer waylays his victim, projecting an aura of heat which stops the victim in his or her tracks. Numbers of *maua* men may "hunt" victims together. If they find a woman in her garden, they call to her from the bush, she goes over, and they copulate with her repeatedly before killing her. Sexuality and sadism are thus closely linked in the *maua* theme. With men, torture of this sort does not occur. The sorcerer simply cuts open the victim's stomach, pulls out the kidneys, places one in the victim's mouth, stuffs the exposed insides with leaves, sews the skin up by magical touch, and sends the person home, telling him or her to cook the kidney and eat it. Where the relatives recognize the signs of *maua*, they will not even at-

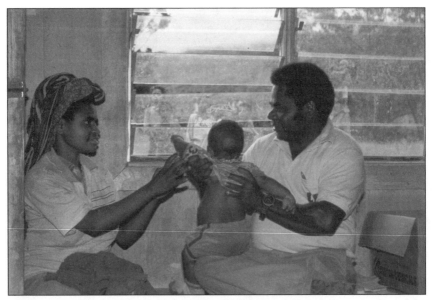

Figure 6–3. A mother presents her child to be examined (Duna).

tempt medical treatment nor is there any indigenous ritual care available. The victim will simply die within the period stated by the sorcerer.

The Wiru have no real equivalent of the general Hagen concept of *popokl*. But they do have very pronounced ideas on the effects of bad feelings on health. Bad feelings are *poanea wene*, and they result from the disruption of proper exchange relationships, in particular when a sister's children fail to make gifts to their mother's people or when their father fails to do so on their behalf and the mother's folk are angry. Sickness results for the sister's children. Payments of wealth must be made to restore them to health. This belief (shared generally with the Hagen people) is very powerfully upheld by the Wiru and forms a constantly invoked cultural symbol of what is correct in social relationships. However, as with the practical workings of ideas concerning the Hagen *popokl*, the Wiru ideas do not exclude western-style health care. Medication will be given; but it is definitely thought that if the proper ritual exchanges are not also made then the sick person cannot recover.

Wiru concepts of sickness and its causation were in the precolonial past centered on religious cults, called *tapa*, *timbu*, and *aroa ipono*, as well as on the "mother's brother" syndrome. These cults are now entirely replaced by Christian sects: the Lutherans, Catholics, Wesleyan, Evangelical Bible Mission, and Church of Christ, and all of those missions also encourage people to use hospitals and aid posts, as well as prayers to God, in their responses to sickness. The Christian religion has therefore slotted in to the place in the scheme of things held by traditional religion previously, while Christianity and biomedicine are seen to be mutually compatible.

Chapter 7

Illness and the Emotions

In considering Ohnuki-Tierney's materials on Japan (Ch. 2), we have noted how she remarks on Japanese physiomorphism, the tendency not to ascribe moral blame in relation to conditions of sickness in the body. However, many personalistic regimens do link illness to social and moral circumstances and moreover tie these in with emotional states. We saw how in Latin American cultures such ideas can apply to the state of *susto*, for example in Mexico (Ch 2). The same pattern has been shown for the Papua New Guinea Highlands (Ch. 6).

We deepen the analysis now with a further case study .

Spiritualist Healers in Mexico

Kaja Finkler has studied the practices of healers in Spiritualist Temples in Mexico in ways that enable us to deepen our understanding of the above point. The Spiritualist movement developed in Mexico in opposition to Catholicism from 1861 onward, and gained influence after 1923 with the building of a head temple in Mexico City and the establishment of a hierarchy of temples attached to it. The head temple is described as the "womb" of the church, and women play an important role in this organization, in contradiction to Catholicism (Finkler 1994a: 15). Thus the head of a temple is often, though not always, a woman, and beneath her are the overseer, the guardian, several "pillars" who watch over the congregations, clairvoyants who testify, the pen of gold functionary, and finally the healers or practitioners, who operate through their putative possession by spirits.

The deities involved in Spiritualist teachings and religious services are those of the Christian religion generally, i.e. God (Jehovah), and Jesus Christ, along with Mother Mary and also Father Elias, the supposed founder of the movement who was the son of an Otomi Indian woman and a *mestizo* father of Spanish-Jewish descent. This founder reputedly added twelve further commandments to the Ten Commandments of the Bible. Services are called irradiations, at which mediums in trance speak God's word directly to the congregation.

109

Spiritualist temples are self-consciously differentiated from Catholic churches. They are devoid of images other than an eye encased in a triangle (this seems equivalent to the Masonic symbol on the U.S. one dollar note). Spiritualists, unlike Catholics, deny the power of witchcraft or the "evil eye." Catholics, in turn, may regard Spiritualists as witches themselves. The healing practices that are integral to the temple's operations are explicitly designed as a mechanism for recruiting persons as temple members, and those who join but subsequently leave are expected to suffer from headaches. Mediums in trance call out the names of dead persons who died in trouble or violence, "giving light" to them and setting them at peace so that they will cease to inflict illness on the living. Healers identify spirits "in the dark" as responsible for particular cases of sickness and invoke spirits of the "high light" as their protectors, who also prescribe medications for the sick. These protectors may be spirits of old Indian healers who lived before the Spanish Conquest or of later personages who prescribe a mixture of herbal and pharmaceutical remedies. Treatment is offered free, but patients are encouraged to join the Temple and to continue to receive the benefits of irradiations. Proper healing is described as *limpio*, making clear, and must conform to the religion's symbolic rules: for example, a medication dosage must be prescribed with an odd number, not an even one (e.g. three drops should be prescribed rather than four). Patients who prove hard to heal are described as "having a gift" and are counseled to turn their afflictions to their advantage by entering into the role of novice healers.

The patients who visit the temples for healing are Mexicans who combine humoral ideas with notions that undesirable emotions can cause sickness (and may themselves be triggered by eating inappropriate foods). Anger is an emotion often cited. Spiritualists incorporate these notions into their own practices, adding the idea that illnesses not curable by physicians can be attributed to perturbed spirits. In deflecting the allocation of blame or responsibility from neighbors, spouses, and kin and in blocking any appeal to the idea of witchcraft by the living, healers emphasize the importance of positive social interactions as a basis for health (Finkler 1994: 53). Healers also specialize in treating those whose disorders appear to be spiritual rather than simply material or physical. They are involved in "correcting" popular and Catholic views of causation and in turning people towards their own religion as a source of healing. Because they do not make competing claims with biomedicine, they are able to offer therapy in a pluralistic market context and in particular they are able to offer services to categories of people who are poor and so cannot afford biomedical treatment, who find it uncomfortable to approach biomedical physicians with certain conditions, and who have chronic, socially-related, health problems that do not yield well to biomedical treatment. These factors apply particularly clearly to women in lower-income households whose lives contain elements of conflict that are difficult to control or manage and whose conditions embody these problems. In these circumstances, while the initial treatment may appear like a cure for a simple disease symptom such as headache or back pain, the longer-term induction into Temple rituals acts as a source of social and spiritual support for habitual or regular patients and serves as a form of psychotherapy for them. Insofar as such patients themselves perceive that they feel better as a result, their treatment can be considered successful even if the underlying disease conditions remain largely the same.

While it is interesting that temple healers profess not to share certain cultural characteristics with their patients, for example by refusing to countenance patients' ideas of witchcraft as a cause of sickness, it is clear that a part of their appeal lies precisely in the sharing of cultural symbols and attitudes, an issue that is always of great importance in doctor-patient interactions. Patients, other than regulars, tend not to seek verbal advice for personal problems, but Finkler acknowledges (p. 61) that the presentation of physical conditions may often be seen as "somatizations of dysphoric affect or other psychological distress." The patient's reluctance to discuss such matters finds comfort in the omniscient role adopted by the healer, putatively by virtue of knowledge gained through trancing and communication with spirits. The patient thus does not need to make an elaborate verbal statement of symptoms or their possible antecedents and concomitants.

Healers appear to be mostly women, although they may be of either sex. They perform healing on Tuesdays and Fridays, and before entering the healing room they approach the altar to hear the temple head pronounce a prayer. They wear a white robe. After entering the healing room they call on their spirit protector to come and settle in their body and identify itself with a greeting for everyone present. The healer then begins to treat patients, helped by an assistant who dispenses aromatic waters. The healer does not show signs of recognizing the patient and confines interactions to impersonal and brief statements conveying authority which appear to mimic in ethos the behavior of biomedical physicians. The healer, however, also exhorts the patient to have faith in the treatment, and exhibits supernatural knowledge that the patient can passively accept. Patients may be comforted by the aura of knowledge and this in turn, Finkler suggests, can act as a "powerful placebo" for them (p. 86).

The healer also performs actions held to be therapeutic. First there is the dislodgement (*desalojo*), referred to by patients as the *limpia*, cleansing. In this the healer lightly massages the patient's body, making tactile contact while keeping eyes closed in trance. Second, the healer asks about the purpose of the visit and probes parts of the body said to be in pain. Sometimes, the healer faints in response to a perceived transference of the evil spirit causing the illness from the patient's body to her own, though patients may not comprehend this event. Finally, the healer prescribes treatments, which involve a wide variety of herbal remedies, usually for teas and baths (e.g. rue, rosemary, balm, camomile, and basil) tonics, tranquilizers, and antidiarrheals, including pharmaceuticals such as milk of magnesia. The healer is usually dogmatic with the patient and may deny a patient's claim to be suffering from, say, *susto* (fright, soul loss), telling the patient there is really nothing wrong. The aromatic waters of ammonia, eau de cologne, or rubbing alcohol, are employed in cleansings. Healers do not enter into family conflicts with advice other than to endure: for example, a wife jealous of a husband's supposed adultery is told simply to make herself nice for him and win him back. Patients who say they are desperate may be told to busy themselves searching for therapeutic flowers and cleansing them for use (p. 90). Finkler gives examples of the 1,212 treatment interactions she observed which strongly reinforce the impression of a hybrid combination of religious symbolism and pragmatic common sense that is probably the formula for success in treatment practices. For example, a young woman has been told to come with branches for a cleansing. The healer divides these into bunches and tells the patient that she is looking at a sacred spirit. The patient reports that her head pain is gone but she is nauseous, and the healer prescribes the juice from three lemons to be taken on three mornings (p. 92). Another patient who had a flower pot fall on his head and reported *susto* as a result was told to make two more visits, bringing flowers, to take baths in water suffused with rosemary and other herbs, and to drink rosemary tea, and was given massage with rubbing alcohol. The healer added: "You lack vitamins. I know everything. Walk on your way smiling" (p. 96).

The reported outcomes of treatment vary according to the status of patients as first-comers, habituals, or regulars. For first-comers and habituals, the rates of success are low except with regard to diarrheas, simple gynecological conditions, and somatizations. Even so, patients return for more treatment quite often. Patients seem in particular to appreciate the cleansings they receive (perhaps by analogy with confession and absolution in Catholicism?). In a chapter entitled "How Spiritualist Healers Heal," Finkler divides the issue of therapeutic events into three components: the doctor-patient relationship, techniques and procedures, and patient characteristics or syndromes (p. 157). By contrast with the biomedical doctor-patient relationship she argues that spiritualist healing depends more on healing techniques than on relationship, and less on shared understandings than on assertion of spiritual power.

The act of cleansing is one of these healing techniques. First, we should note that the healers call it "dislodging," which seems to refer to the removal of a malign spirit from the patient's body, a highly "personalistic" image in Foster's terms (see Ch. 2). The patients, in calling it a cleansing, a "making clear," seem to be appealing to another side of the imagery of dark (spirits) versus (spirits of) light, one set in "naturalistic" terms. The two forms of imagery may arguably be said to complement each other rather than indicate a lack of shared concepts. Whether this is so or not, we can agree with Finkler's own point, that cleansing suggests a symbolic termination of the patient's sick role, enabling the patient to adopt, at least for a while, the role of a person who is well. Finkler also points out here that the observation applies best to first-comers and habitual patients, whereas for regulars the sick role is not so much terminated as re-framed, when the patient becomes herself inducted as a healer (p. 163) and also experiences trancing which may have mildly beneficial effects.

A second technique is the tactile communication, which probably relaxes patients and may induce mild trancing and responsiveness to what the healer says. For regulars the ritual "technique" of irradiation may act symbolically to stimulate pain-reducing endorpins in the body, giving relief from symptoms in a way that corresponds to the well-known placebo effect (p. 168). On the other hand, participation in temple rituals can also bring on feelings of guilt and anxiety about not being obedient enough to the will of spirits. (There are parallels here with fundamentalist Christianity.) The overall function here is social, not medical: to bind regulars further to the temple itself. This is done partly through the deployment of images, as in the case of one woman, Chucha, who was told that her heart palpitations were like crystalline drops falling into a glass and these in turn were like God's words entering into (and fertilizing?) Chucha during irradiations. Images of purity and purification seem important, and Finkler links this theme to the idea of corruption and struggle in Mexico's history and the desire to be cleansed and renewed.

This set of techniques works well with regulars who have only mild conditions of a kind we might recognize as psychiatric. It does not work for more severe cases, such as Concha (p. 179), whose mother thought that she had been "bewitched by her father's girlfriend, who had deliberately fed the girl food that had brought on her condition." As Concha failed to respond to Spiritualist ministrations the mother became desperate and more convinced than ever that her condition was due to witchcraft. Finkler comments that even to a casual observer Concha's condition was "generalized schizophrenia," a severe psychosis (p. 179). Contrast Concha's case with that of Pancho, a wealthy middle-aged man who suffered from severe pain in the lumbar region and was prescribed surgery by a physician. A temple healer placed a shawl around his waist and pulled it forcibly from side to side. His pain disappeared. One might call this a lucky chiropractic strike (p. 136). Of such contradictory stuff are medical outcomes made.

Curing and Healing

Finkler calls the temple practitioners healers, but she also sometimes refers to them as curers, implying that she uses the two terms interchangeably. From our viewpoint it is worthwhile to make some distinctions. In the pragmatic sense, what the practitioners are doing most of the time is attempting to cure particular conditions. Their prescriptions are very like European folk-medicine and perhaps overlap with those of *curandero* or *curandera*, male or female popular practitioners. In this regard, they seem to have patchy success, but offer a partial, culturally appealing alternative to biomedicine in a pluralistic context. In the symbolic sense, however, what they are attempting to do is to heal, to restore a sense of wellbeing in the patient as a person by offering her/him a renewed sense of personhood. This is done by the healing techniques described and can be seen also as a ritual alternative to the Catholic religion. We can go further and say that these techniques actually establish a doctor-patient relationship, albeit not like an individual, biomedical doctor-patient relationship. This goal of healing is shown most clearly with regulars who have chronic, mild somatized or psychiatric conditions. For these, healing in the sense of being given a renewed sense of life as a whole most clearly takes place, even though they may not be cured of some disease they have. In the typical therapeutic interaction, however, we are witnessing a hybrid curing/healing performance in which cleansing represents the healing part and the prescription the curing part. In this case, as in others, understanding why a particular combination of curing and healing elements occurs depends on seeing how medical practices fit into wider contexts of the society, both in terms of basic cultural ideas and in terms of historical changes and power conflicts that accompany such changes.

Finkler's study raises at a number of turns the question of psychological factors, especially in conditions seen as somatized. A whole branch of medical anthropology is concerned with this kind of question, which we examine next.

Chapter 8

Ethnopsychiatry

Aboriginal Australia

Studies in medical anthropology by psychiatrists are usually identifiable because of their continuing use of psychiatric theory as cross-culturally acceptable. This is true of John Cawte's book "Medicine is the Law" (Cawte 1974). Cawte's major point is contained in the book's title: that Australian Aboriginal curers or doctors play a big role in social control within their communities; medicine and the law are continuously working together. This situation resembles that among the Huli people as described by Frankel (see Ch. 6, Medical Pluralism), in respect to sicknesses where spirits or God are held to be responsible. Also, running through this major argument, is the psychiatric thread. For example, when Cawte discusses Walbiri (Aboriginal Australian) medicine, he refers to the concept of *millelba*, a spirit counterpart who generally watches over a person but causes sickness in cases when there has been wrongdoing. Cawte compares this to Freud's concept of motivational meaning as expressed in his "Studies on Hysteria" (p. 34).

He refers also to Freud's concept of transference. Patients transfer to their physicians attitudes they had to parents and other authority figures that they put their faith in. So Aboriginal healers must depend on that trust or faith also. But culture change fragments communities and people's ideas, and makes it harder for the healer to successfully work. To be effective, the healer must know the individuals and their histories. The Aboriginal Walbiri doctors in the North Kimberley area of Western Australia are not persons who have healed themselves of sickness, as shamans are commonly said to be. They are under pressure from mission health personnel, who sometimes regard them as heathens and interferers. The Walbiri doctors themselves say their *mabanba*, healing spirit, is weakened by white man's medicine. In interpreting illness, they may say it is caused by *millelba* or by *tjanba*, punishing spirits, or possession of *mamul* spirits, or *yarda* sorcery, in which solid objects are projected into people's bodies. The *mabanba* familiar can fly out and look for the source of sorcery that has been made against a sick person. "*Mabanba* embodies the omnipotence of doctors, as the object psychology of the people requires" (p. 47). *Mamul* spirits attack a victim's kidney fat (see below), which then has to be replaced by the Walbiri doctor. Poison sticks of mulga tree wood are used to sing *yarda* sorcery into people. Fear of such sorcery causes a high level of anxiety. The role of *tjanba* is played by human dancers, decorated as the *tjanba* spirit, and appointed to carry out an execution by the elders. Cawte recognizes (p. 53) superego and id functions in these representations. He attempts to match or merge Freudian concepts to his ethnographic data, and this attempt becomes largely an exercise in historical plausibility or the juxtaposition of data with psychological interpretation. Here he simply asserts that solid objects used in magic do correspond to these Freudian categories.

Tjagolo are magical objects that can cause harm, previously used between political groups. Belief in and use of such objects was declining when Cawte conducted his research, but *tjimi* beliefs were flourishing. *Tjimi* were gremlins, becoming equated with the Devil through Christian teaching and capable of being blamed for untoward events. Indigenous specialists gain their power through a lifelong association with Ungur, the mythical Serpent. *Tjagolo*, in fact, are analogous with the Serpent's eggs which enter the doctor's navel during his initiation (p. 64). Ungur gives the doctor the power to remove such *tjagolo* from others.

Cawte discusses a number of individual victims of sorcery whom he thought to be suffering from paranoid schizophrenia, pathological personality, depressive state, hypochondriasis, organic brain deterioration, and carcinoma. The questions that arise in relation to all this are: (1) are these descriptions intended to suggest that the ideas about sorcery have in the first place originated with such individuals? (2) if so, how? (3) If not, what about the cases of other victims who were not psychotic, etc.? For example, the paranoid schizophrenic who heard spirits talking to him also blamed his condition on excrement sorcery (i.e. sorcery carried out on his stolen feces). Would all victims of such sorcery be mentally unbalanced or not? Another Kaiadilt man in the group Cawte was working with, in his forties, had suffered physical and social dislocation and was depressed. He expressed this by saying that he too had suffered from excrement sorcery. Cawte comments that the man's social circumstances were sufficient to explain his depression. What, then, would be the function of the explanation in terms of sorcery? Cawte fails to take the opportunity to tackle this question. He remarks (p. 101): "Those basic values we call mental health are not really so ethnocentric as some would have us believe. They are exemplified in such an institution as sorcery. It is an ancient or exotic syndrome, but fashioned of the universal stuff of mental health — personal comfort and social efficiency!"

Cawte traces the high incidence of mental sickness to contact with Europeans. He considers the Yowera area of Australia, inhabited by some 700+ people in the 1960's, and describes several cases of highly abnormal behavior, each associated with some traditional belief but marked by schizoid and/or catatonic symptoms. The traditional belief content is that spirit animals have lodged in the body (e.g., rainbow serpent, fish). These can be personal "totems" transmitted by practitioners to their sons. Here Cawte moves into a full-blown psychiatric explanation: the father, a tribal, interpreted his trouble as a spirit inside himself, i.e., mania in clinical terms; the sons split it off as something outside, i.e., schizophrenia (p. 181). This analysis suggests schizophrenia as a culture-contact syndrome. Cawte gives a number of other cases of disturbance, and refers to "the crisis of Aboriginal identity, the resistance to whites, the disturbance of domesticity associated with poverty, the social fragmentation, and the pervasive deprivation." We can see many of the cases he describes as resulting from an unfortunate collapse of cultural patterns, leading not to a kind of pluralism but to a veritable crisis of personality management. Anxiety is the result.

A different approach is provided by Janice Read in "Sorcerers and Healing Spirits." Her ethnographic materials partially overlap with Cawte's but her treatment is monographic, and she does not use Freudian categories for her analysis, being concerned with culture, social structure, and history. She deals with the Yolngu people at Yirrkala, otherwise known as the Murngin and first studied by Lloyd Warner, subsequently also by Nancy Williams and by Ian Keen. These people, in the Northern Territory of Australia, were also visited by Cawte during his survey work. Like other Aborigines, the Yolngu people valued their traditional lands greatly but had lost most of them and lived in settlements around government and mission services. During the 1970s a reverse process of out-migration also took place. Yirrkala itself was a small town with about 800 Aborigines living there, mostly living off mining royalties. The living environment was not hygienic — bad water and sewage arrangements led to gastrointestinal disease and hookworm, with anemia, eye infections, and skin diseases. Respiratory tract infections were also common and sleeping arrangements were crowded in wet weather. Alcohol consumption was a problem, too. Reid's major argument is that the handling of sickness is not to be seen as an isolated subsystem of behavior, because it enables these people to maintain some prediction over events in their own lives, a control which their subjugation within white society has historically removed from them in other ways.

From this account, it is clear that the idea that sickness comes from the actions of sorcerers and spirits is very much alive at Yirrkala. In this relatively egalitarian Aboriginal society, jealousy is held to result in sorcery against the resented person, but at the same time sorcery accusations are not ordinarily made within the community — a contradiction, because jealousy certainly does operate *within* the community and not between strangers. This kind of fear and jealousy is projected into white society also: an indigenous *marrngitj* (healer) said he was afraid to accept an invitation from a white doctor to work at a hospital with him because the other white doctor would be jealous and hurt him.

Sacred places may also be places of danger where people can contract illness, especially if they transgress ritual prohibitions, i.e., not to gather food in such areas. This is just an example of food-related restrictions. For example, during pregnancy women should not eat foods with "totemic" associations, for these may cause abnormalities.

The marriage system also precipitates sickness, in the sense that wrong marriages are held to result in illness. The connecting link is anger. If young bethrothed women reject their betrothed and go to a lover instead, there is anger and sorcery may result later. The people recognize that disturbance in social relationships is then the "cultural" cause of rates of sickness. Sorcery is the proximate cause, the instrument.

Yolngu distinguish between the healer and the sorcerer. The healer's role is well defined. Healers become so through a "supernatural" experience which makes them "clever." Such an ability has to be demonstrated by practical healing. Sprits are held to give these men healing stones. Reid quotes an informant's story of this process, (pp. 59–61). One stone this man had was an "x-ray" stone which enabled him to see inside a patient's body. Adults of either sex, and children, can practice as healers. Despite their contacts with the supernatural, healers are not psychologically abnormal. Sometimes, doubts are expressed about them. Their main task is to combat the effects of sorcery, *galka*, and this is held to be not easy. Reid notes that the healer functions also as a doctor, a therapist, and a priest, so the role is complex and demanding (p. 78).

The account by a healer of how he acquired his powers indicates that he was concerned, somewhat, to know whether the spirits that visited him were caused by *galka* sorcery or not. This in itself indicates an area of ambiguity between the "good" healer and the "bad" sorcerer. The healer, in fact, may sometimes be feared also as a sorcerer. There are many parallels to this idea in ethnographic accounts. What is striking is that the Yolngu are concerned to deny the ambiguity. This tendency may be reinforced by historical change. *Galka* are associated with the pagan past. On at least one level the Yolngu are Christians, and they can allow themselves to keep their healers more easily than their sorcerers. However, at least one case history also shows the conflict between the missions and indigenous healers, in which the mission workers argue that people must choose only Jesus—a demand that runs counter to the grain of eclecticism which is the usual response of people when faced with more than one system of beliefs.

The *Galka* is one who attacks the body and destroys its blood; the *Marrngitj* is the one who can set the blood to rights without hurting the body's organs further. In either case, as Reid says (p. 79), it is the vulnerability of the body that is in focus. Blood, also, is a focus of power, which may be either beneficial or harmful, depending on whether it is controlled or not. Sick people fear the loss of blood or that their blood will be "finished" (this is exactly the same as the Melpa idea). In rituals of purification and liberation of patients or of persons who have been at a funeral, sometimes red ochre is used to symbolize "the blood which was lost" and to restore strength (p. 81).

The *galka* extracts blood, and this will result in death, unless he aborts his work. In one case a *galka* is said to have recognized a woman as his relative and therefore to have thrown some of her blood into a lake, thus cooling his magic, rather than burying it for later use. This alone enabled her to survive. This image of the sorcerer as cutter and breacher of boundaries explains attitudes to surgery: the surgeon is seen somewhat as the *galka* is. Surgery is held to waste the body and spoil the blood. One man who was operated on wanted Reid to ask the Department of Health for compensation for his loss of blood! The sorcerer may use heat also to dry up body essences (such as urine, feces, sweat). Heat is inimical, too, to healing. One child healer who lost interest in healing was said by his parents to have drunk too much hot tea. Underpants of a person may be taken and stuffed into car exhausts. When the engine starts its heat will cause the person sickness in the pelvic region.

Another substance that *galka* take in addition to blood is fat. Fat is a major indicator of life and life force is often thought to be transferred through it. In humans and other animals kidney fat is especially significant, and some sorcerers are said to specialize in stealing people's kidney fat. The inevitable result for the victim is death.

The *marrngitj's* job in Reid's study is to restore the body to health against the noxious effects of disease. As we have noted, people are loath to accuse community members of sorcery. They deny that there are *galka* among them. However, in 1981, they were more willing to admit to the anthropologist that sorcerers were closer to home than they had been in 1974. Blaming an outside *galka* can reflect a desire to remove blame from inside the community, e.g., if a man fights and kills a kinsman he may be said to have been told by a *galka* from outside to do this (p. 88). Clans are corporately vulnerable to revenge attacks. They try to keep marriage within certain alliances, because if outsider women are married they may become vehicles for sorcery. Reid sums up (p. 90): "The sorcerer and healer personify the polarities in Yolngu concepts of social order and security: conflict and harmony, sickness and health, danger and safety, outside and inside." This in itself gives one clue to an answer to the question: how is it that the indigenous system of meanings regarding sickness is adhered to after "a half century of change"? Old ideas have been ingeniously extended to the situation of new problems, she notes (p. 119).

Where western teaching and the teaching of the Aboriginal elders are in conflict, individuals can either ignore the contradictions, live with them, or else synthesize. Different solutions are arrived at by (a) professed Christians, (b) health workers, and (c) young people in general. Nevertheless, even the health workers were all convinced of the dangers of sorcery. Symptoms of sorcery *don't show* in biomedical tests, but patients die, they say (exactly the same idea syndrome as in Papua New Guinea). Especially if a death is sudden or untoward they think of *galka*.

Young Christians educated in Bible College sometimes cite worry as a cause of illness - a view that community members also accept. But this does not preclude suspicion that sorcery may also be involved in some cases. Use of a *marrngitj* can be rationalized by suggesting that maybe God gives the indigenous healer power to cure sickness. Pentecostal revivals passed through Arnhem Land in the late 1970s and until 1981, leaving the people rather serious about God, but still they attempt to put together their traditional beliefs with the new doctrines. Equally, there are skeptics who say they don't believe in sorcery but are not Christians (pp. 132–3). The same death may be made subject to different explanations, e.g., *galka* or battery acid. Alcohol may be blamed, but sorcery also suspected by close kin. Individual variability leads to reverse reasoning: not everyone dies of this, so.... The stories of concern following the deaths of heavy drinkers are tragic, indeed. It is clear also that there is cultural conflict and much confusion — there is no easy syncretism or integration of ideas. Reid emphasizes (p. 153) there is a use of western medicine for treatment, but adherence to Yolngu ideas for explanation—a kind of syncretic compartmentalization of practice versus ideas. There is also an interesting indication that dispersal to homelands *does* lead to better health, away from Yirrkala itself. In general, the sociomedical theory continues to apply because it is sufficiently adaptive to and backed by experience (p. 156).

The examples from Aboriginal Australia we have discussed so far in this chapter indicate how broad the range of materials is that may be encompassed under the heading of ethnopsychiatry. We started from the viewpoint that ethnopsychiatry sometimes depends on western psychiatry for its theoretical background, but the ethnographic materials soon took us into general discussions of ideas and practices about sorcery. Emotions, such as anger, are clearly involved, as we have found in chapter seven on illness and the emotions. In the remainder of this chapter we reconsider the scope of the ethnopsychiatric approach, taking our cues from the work of Atwood Gaines (1992).

Gaines takes his own stance from a position that is prevalent in American anthropology: all systems are culturally constructed and their construction can be studied ethnographically. At the same time it grounds itself in the special study of a class of phenomena that can be called psychiatric, i.e. the treatment of forms of mental derangement, considered cross-culturally. Professional western psychiatry is studied along with other forms of folk and professional psychiatries around the world. The analytical focus is on interpretation, understanding the logic and orientation of the system in question. This kind of approach precludes the uncritical use of western theory as an underlying guide to analysis. We found this approach both exemplified in Cawte's work on Australian Aborigines and implicitly opposed by Janice Read's work on the Yolngu of Arnhem Land. Gaines points out here that if behavioral normality is culturally constructed, so must be abnormality (1992:8). Ethnopsychiatry needs to take both normality and abnormality into account and therefore must bridge over into a consideration of social personhood, the self, and relations with others, matters that are in fact crucially symbolised in areas such as ideas about sorcery and witchcraft and their relationship to moral ideals. At this point ethnopsychiatry ceases again to be a bounded domain and begins to overlap with other topical foci in medical anthropology, for example embodiment theory.

The implicitly culturalist and relativist outlook exemplified in Gaines' exposition is one which he also contrasts with approaches in critical medical anthropology (CMA, see Ch. 13 of this book). Authors of these approaches are said to attribute the causes of sickness to entities such as capitalism or the state, whereas such concepts, according to Gaines, are ethnocentric creations of these authors themselves, based on theories of universalism, and "ignoring culture, history, meaning and human agency" (p. 19). Gaines outlines some key assumptions that inform his own cultural constructivist approach: (1) medical knowledge is problematic, and biomedicine itself encompasses many local traditions (see also chapter six in this book, on medical pluralism); (2) ethnomedical realities are created through social interactions. This applies to the discourse of biomedical specialists as much as to debates about divination, sorcery, and witchcraft; (3) ethnomedical systems are open-ended products of cultural history and are consequently in processes of change; (4) ethnomedicine is an expression of culture, as Ohnuki-Tierney shows for Japanese biomedicine (see chapter two); and (5) ethnomedicine has to do with human experiential realities (such as we discuss in chapter nine on religious healing).

Most aspects of this programmatic statement can be found implicitly embedded in one or another part of the present book, as we have just indicated. However, it is worthwhile perhaps to state that we do not espouse the ethnopsychiatric approach in such sharp opposition to critical medical anthropology as Gaines does. Rather, we think that these partially opposed viewpoints are probably compatible in wider schemes of analysis and may have useful things to learn from each other (see Ch. 13).

There is also the problem inherent in all culturally relativist positions of how to achieve comparisons between systems putatively based on unique forms of cultural logic. In practice cultural logics may show overlap or similarity; while if they show difference, we need to find ways to explain the difference as well as to understand what it is, and the search for explanation may lead us to material, historical, and economic causes. For example, we have mentioned sorcery and witchcraft beliefs. While these may be seen as resulting from purely cultural ways of constructing the world, we can also see them as being exacerbated by conditions of ecological stress and by historical movements of people (Riebe 1987). Alterations in political space may also be involved (Stewart and Strathern 1997), as we have noted too.

There are two further arenas in which the ethnopsychiatric approach is regularly put to the test. One is in the definition of the "mentally abnormal." It is clearly straightforward to point out that what is considered abnormal in one cultural context may be seen as quite normal in another; correlatively that standards of, e.g., sanity have to be constructed locally (see for example Nuckolls' study comparing South Indian shamanic and American psychiatric diagnoses, in Gaines 1992: 69–84). It is more difficult, perhaps, to delineate a sphere of "the mental" as such in which the abnormal or normal can be identified, since the mind/body continuum or relationship is itself assessed differently in different cultural traditions (see e.g. A.J. Strathern 1996 on this problem). Hence ethnopsychiatry cannot itself rest unproblematically on concepts of the mind. Conditions that we may attribute to mental abnormality may be thought of by others as cases of spirit possession, for example.

This problem is related to the well-known issue of "culture-bound syndromes" that turns up here. Are there special forms of illness peculiar to certain cultures and describable only in their own terms? In a sense the logic of cultural constructionism forces us to say that at a certain level *every* illness within a cultural repertoire is particular to that culture. But this would not preclude us from, again, recognizing similarities and overlaps; and in practice attention has tended to focus on syndromes that clearly appear to have distinctive features.

Well-known examples are *amok* (aggressive) behavior and *latah* (startle complex), both found in Southeast Asia. Both could be seen as elaborations of much more widely, if not universally, found behavioral tendencies. For example, *popokl* anger among the Melpa of Mount Hagen in Papua New Guinea may lead to aggressive behavior, but it is *also* thought to cause sickness in the person who experiences it, so as a syndrome it is quite different from *amok*: nevertheless, one could argue that *popokl is* itself a culture-bound syndrome. Further, startling another person, called *ropa rut ndui*, is held in classic fashion to dislodge the *min* or spirit from its connection with the body and therefore to make a person behave oddly, but without the elaboration of *latah*.) We choose here for discussion a less well-known example, labeled "Parsitis" (Pliskin 1987), in a study of "cultural constraints on sickness and diagnosis of Iranians in Israel."

This diagnosis arises in a classic situation of cultural pluralism. It also emerges in an equally classic context of personal and geographic displacement, so that, properly understood it could simply be called "displacement illness" and would be found to be increasingly prevalent in a mobile world of migrants and refugees. Pliskin notes (p. 192) that "when Iranians, as patients, express in very Iranian ways bodily problems to Israeli clinicians who cannot discover any pathological basis for their complaints," the physicians label the condition "Parsitis." (It could also be called simply "other-itis.") The syndrome corresponds to what Arthur Kleinman first identified as "somatization" (also discussed in the work on Japan by Ohnuki-Tierney). The clinician needs a label in order to establish a course of treatment, and the patient also seeks to have a name for the condition experienced as well as a legitimation of it (we can compare the problem of "chronic fatigue syndrome," CFS, and how it is viewed by patients and clinicians). Such labels may be influenced by cultural models or by ones of social class, Pliskin points out: behavior classified as mental illness among lower-class people may be seen as personal peculiarities among those of the upper class (p. 195).

In the context Pliskin is describing, some of the physicians did not recognize somatized conditions (such as Parsitis) to be legitimate symptoms of distress, so did not refer them to psychiatric workers. Some patients shunned the psychiatric clinic because of stigma. The physical symptoms exhibited/reported were headaches, weakness, backaches, overall pain, palpitations, no appetite, dizziness, insomnia, stomach ache, indigestion, arm or leg pain, rheumatism , and "liver burning." These patients revealed also fear, anger, and suppression of negative feelings, worry, impotence, and the like. Most were eventually diagnosed psychiatrically with varieties of depression. They did not themselves talk about feelings or emotions, however, but reported their bodily conditions in the somatizing manner. Pliskin comments: "Israeli clinicians speak about the similarities of Iranian patients as opposed to other patients, seeing them as somatizers with strange bodily complaints who cannot function in their work or familial roles" (p. 201).The label Parsitis thus becomes an informal diagnostic entity, functioning on the basis of a stereotype, and leading to further possibilities of misdiagnosis. At the back of this situation is the Iranian concept of *narahati*, or sadness associated with being away from home.

Iranians tended, however, not to reveal such sadness since it indicates vulnerability and powerlessness. Instead, therefore, they referred to a wide range of bodily symptoms, including some that are also culturally influenced, for example "liver burning"or "lack of blood" (concepts incidentally that would be quite amenable to being understood by Papua New Guinean peoples such as the Melpa of Mount Hagen. See Chapter 3). Pliskin gives a detailed account of several case histories to substantiate her point and concludes that culture is crucially involved in all clinical transactions and intercultural problems of misunderstanding develop which give rise to what Pliskin calls "silent boundaries" between clinician and patient.

Pliskin's study is highly relevant to several of our themes in this book, such as medical pluralism and doctor-patient communication (Chapters 6 and 12). Its significance for the issue of "culture-bound syndromes" is that it shows how the kind of labeling arises in clinical encounters that leads to the invention of a pseudo-category, a misdiagnosed culture-bound syndrome that is really a product of interethnic misunderstandings. Such a phenomenon is clearly different from, for example, *latah*, in which the stereotyping of behavioral repertoires takes place by mutual agreement within a cultural arena, not by misunderstanding across such arenas. Nevertheless, the phenomenon of labeling, and its amplifying effect, is found in both intra- and inter-cultural contexts. Furthermore, Iranian Parsitis is also understandable in cross-cultural terms as a form of reaction to geographical and social displacement, and, as we have noted, that is a syndrome which is far from being peculiar to the "Iranians in Israel" situation.

Our general point here is that while from one viewpoint culture-bound syndromes are perfectly real, from other viewpoints the concept is of less value, since it may lead us to ignore similarities and essentialize differences. Ethnopsychiatry does not need, therefore, to depend on this concept as one of its major ways of understanding the world, even if the discipline does stress the importance of different cultural logics. Somatization, for instance, following the work of Kleinman, is recognized as a phenomenon that occurs widely in many cultural contexts, including everyday contexts in Britain and the USA as well as in China, New Guinea, and among Iranians in Israel.

Pliskin's study also reveals the morally evaluative dimensions of communication that may underline patterns of doctor-patient interaction. The Iranian patients made their own evaluations of themselves and were constrained by a morality of strength versus weakness. The Israeli clinicians, on the other hand, saw the patients' failure to talk about their familial or social problems as marks of their failure to perform morally in their roles. Paul Brodwin's study of "medicine and morality" in Haiti (Brodwin 1996) shows very clearly how moral status is at issue in situations of illness, influenced by Catholicism. Haitians have developed a Manichaean picture of the human person (which is now beginning to show also in places like Mount Hagen in Papua New Guinea), based on the ethnotheory of the good soul and the bad soul. Catholic herbalists invoke the help of good angels that come to them in dreams and show them how to treat their patients, and claim that sickness itself is sent by Satanic forces known as *lwa* and invoked by people who wish maliciously to hurt others, their enemies, and therefore consult *houngan* (indigenous forms of ritual specialists). Sickness itself may be seen, then, as a result of the enmity of others (see, for example, cases in Brodwin 1996: 182). It is in the curing of sickness that moral contests occur which then turn the curing into healing, an encounter between the good and the bad that is supposed to reaffirm the social values of morality as seen in the image of the good angel. Brodwin's study shows that forms of frenzied behavior, interpreted as possession by dead spirits and reflecting stressful situations in life, are also treated in a religious framework, since they are seen as displacing temporarily the person's "good spirit" and healing is needed to drive out the bad spirit and bring the good one back (p. 183). Brodwin's study indicates both the truth in ethnopsychiatry's basic standpoint that local cultural logics must be understood and the difficulty in combining this with a model of "mental" abnormality, since this abnormality may be experienced and expressed in Haiti as spirit possession. We will look at this problem further in the next chapter, which deals with healing in a context of charismatic Catholicism, not in Haiti but in the United States of America.

Chapter 9

Spiritual Healing: Charismatic Catholics

Thomas Csordas is a cultural anthropologist who has studied the phenomenon of the Charismatic Catholic Renewal and its emphasis on healing since 1973. The Renewal is a movement that explicitly incorporates Pentecostal-style practices into Catholic ritual. Pentecostal practices stress speaking in tongues (hence their name), inspiration from the Holy Spirit, and the healing of the sick by means of prayers and the invocation of divine power. The Catholic Renewal began in 1967 in the United States when a set of faculty members of Duquesne University in Pittsburgh, who had undergone the experience of conversion to Pentecostal ways, decided to bring these into the Catholic Church rather than leaving it and joining a Pentecostal congregation (Shaara 1994: 109; Csordas 1994: 16; 1997: 4). The movement was facilitated by the liberalizing of Catholic liturgy that followed the pronouncements of the Second Vatican Council. It promises to its members a "personal relationship" with Jesus and access to "spiritual gifts" through charisma (Csordas, p. 18). Both of these features are exactly the same as leading motifs in charismatic Protestant churches of Pentecostal-style derivation such as the Assemblies of God churches, whose members in Mount Hagen, Papua New Guinea, explained these matters to us on our fieldwork visits in 1997 and 1998. But Charismatic Catholics, rather than using the imagery of being "born again" as many Pentecostalists do, rather say they have discovered their "real self"; which explains the title of Csorda's book, "The Sacred Self," since the real self is the one that is sacred in the sense of being "who I am in Christ" (Csordas, ibid.). Csordas further identifies themes to do with spontaneity, control, and intimacy as involved in the celebration of this idea of the sacred self, themes he relates to North American culture generally. The overall theme of "health" in turn comes to stand for the proper arrangement of all these factors in life. Ritual healing conduces toward this state, so that "to be healed is to inhabit the Charismatic world as a sacred self" (Csordas, p. 24). And to reach this state the self involved must first be "wounded" or "broken" as a prelude to being healed.

The overall question that Csordas seeks to answer at the beginning of the book is one that has been asked many times: "How does religious healing work, if indeed it does?"(p. 1). The answers to this question depend greatly on what meanings are given to the term "healing" itself. They are therefore also central, in a larger sense, to the major theme of this book, the distinction between curing and healing. Whatever the specifics of its meanings in different contexts, healing in our usage, as in Csordas's, refers always to the person seen as a totality; whereas curing refers primarily to specific conditions that a person may be experiencing. In his study, Csordas wished to show how religious healing worked for the holistic "selves" of the people he was investigating. The sacred self is the self that has been healed, or made whole, since it has been brought into harmony with God.

In addition, however, Charismatics practice specific rituals of healing. These began with a spontaneous event in 1974 at the Notre Dame football stadium during the movement's annual conference, when healing is said to have "broken out unexpectedly." This is classic for Pentecostal-style narratives, in which beginnings are depicted as coming in a rush of the spirit that sweeps people into itself like the original descent of cloven tongues of fire on the Apostles of Jesus. In the routinized services that followed the 1974 canonical event, a healing minister officiates, ushers receive people coming forward for prayers, "catchers" are ready for those who swoon when overwhelmed by divine power, and there are also musicians and small prayer teams (Csordas 1994: 36). Participants come forward for the Eucharist, are anointed with oil, experience a laying on of hands by the minister, and are prayed over. The healers may ask people to name their problem, announce it themselves by inspiration, or "leave everything to God." Sometimes the priest holds healing sessions in a special room where prayer teams also spend a longer time with supplicants, and these in turn may be followed by further, more lengthy private sessions that consist of both counseling and healing prayer. Healing prayer can also be practiced in solitude. The ability to heal is considered one of the spiritual gifts that come with charisma. It may involve the ability to discern the presence of evil spirits and to exorcize them.

The healers distinguish between the physical healing of the body, the inner healing of emotional distress, and deliverance from evil spirits. The first category corresponds to what we call curing (physical healing), though its techniques are obviously different from those of biomedicine; inner healing is consonant with our general category of healing as such. There seems to be quite a stress on inner healing, seen as both the healing of relationships and the healing of memories. Interestingly, some Pentecostalists reject this form of healing on the grounds that Jesus confined himself to physical healing; yet the rhetoric of Pentecostalism is full of expressions that imply that inner healing is the result of finding Jesus and being saved. Demons can be cast out only by priests using the full ritual of exorcism, and it is thought that God then compels the demons to leave, although they may utter curses through the mouths of those they have possessed (p. 410).

A fairly elaborate body of ideas has developed around these practices. For example, physical illness may be said to result from biographical trauma and therefore inner healing is needed before physical healing can proceed; or an affliction by evil spirits is said to result from vulnerability caused by a previous traumatic event. A physical condition may be said to have social causes, for example arthritis can be attributed to resentment over having been wronged. The patient is then asked to forgive the offender and prayers are made for inner healing before physical healing is sought. The parallels with Mt. Hagen ideas of *popokl* (anger, frustration, resentment) are very clear (see Chapter 3). A number of clearly designated performance acts correspond to the various areas of healing. "Calling down the blood of the Lamb," for example, is done to protect the supplicant while the "binding of spirits" is for deliverance. The healer experiences "the anointing" when empowered to carry out a healing act through the workings of the Spirit on his/her own spirit at a "deep level." The "laying on of hands" is a gesture or act expressing both intimacy and control, and may also take the form of "therapeutic touch," which consists of moving the hands over the bodies of worshippers in Christ, creating what Csordas, following an innovative formulation by the anthropologist John Blacking, calls a state of *protoritual* (Csordas 1994: 56, quoting Blacking 1977: 14). Protoritual is defined as a state of collective being from which co-ordinated forms of ritual appear to flow spontaneously, very much as in Pentecostalists' own description of being "moved by the Spirit." Protoritual in this sense is thus a constituent part of what Csordas calls the experience of healing.

Csordas's most important argument, which is in fact the basis for his book (Csordas 1994: viii), is that the healings which ministers perform are basically seen as *self processes*. By this phrase he means that the supplicant or patient is involved in making the changes necessary to healing, and through the healer's intervention is enabled to achieve this by divine empowerment. Thus physical healing is said to occur to the individual spontaneously, just as protoritual is said to occur spontaneously at the collective level. Healing is an alteration in the *somatic mode of attention* (Csordas 1994: 67), that is, in the orientation of the embodied self towards the world. The therapeutic process entails an alteration of this kind and is an alteration in the process of "making the self" over time. The efficacy of the ritual healing thus has to be seen in the light of this proposition.

In one case, a fifty-six-year-old married male academic with a Ph.D in biology had been suffering increasingly from attacks of severe backache for many years without seeking biomedical attention for them. He belonged to the Charismatic movement and underwent a healing session at which he felt a purely spiritual experience, but afterwards his back was much better. Thereafter, even when he experienced the beginnings of an attack he would thank God for having cured him, and the attack would be only minor. He reported that he could even shovel snow (Csordas's research was conducted mostly in New England). Csordas rejects explanations of this man's condition as "psychosomatic" and of his healing as by "suggestion." Rather, he says, the man's somatic attention changed and he was alert to his problem, so that he could handle it. The condition is one from which many people suffer. We can suggest that it was at least exacerbated by tension, and when the sufferer consciously relaxed, remembering his healing, the attacks were milder and his overall cyclical state of being prone to them was ameliorated (Csordas 1994: 69). What is involved is incremental efficacy rather than miracle healings, but the "experience of the sacred" is an integral part of the incremental process.

The stress on incremental change here may be somewhat specific to the Catholic Charismatic groups Csordas studied, but he suggests that processes of an incremental kind may in fact underlie the practices of healing in other religious systems as well. Further, healing itself is seen as a necessary prelude to achieving a full life in the religious community. "More precisely.... the sacred self is created as a member of that collectivity defined as the kingdom of God" (Csordas 1994: 160).

One of the mechanisms whereby healing is said to occur is through the production of images, which can be manipulated to enact healing performances. In one session, the healer invited the patient to visualize the liturgical chalice (the cup of holy communion) and to put herself as a little child and then her parents into the cup, and place all her bitterness, anger, resentment, and hate also into the cup, offering it all to Jesus. The healer asked the patient what she then saw, and she answered that she saw Jesus open his arms to receive her and the cup was poured out. She saw also the Blessed Mother (the Virgin Mary) and then Jesus said to her "You have our hearts." The fusion of the woman as a child with herself was said to make her "feel more grown up" and helped her to overcome the hatred of her father which was felt when she remembered how he had abused her as a child (Csordas 1994: 128–129).

Csordas calls sequences like this "imaginal performances." Here the event was characterized also by the "revelatory retrieval of memories," that were then placed into the cup containing the blood of Jesus. The healer further asked the patient to put herself and her husband into the paten (the plate that holds the body of Christ) and to offer this also to Jesus. In a sense the whole problem was placed in the hands of Jesus by this imagined act, and we can say that the persons involved themselves became sacrificial offerings to Jesus, mingled with his own sacred body and blood that are seen as the source of salvation. At a crucial point the healer asked "Is the Lord near?" because empowerment comes only when the deity approaches. And as a supportive background for the whole ritual, helpers prayed energetically in tongues, thereby creating a mystical aura of energy and beseeching the deity to draw near. The chief image, the chalice itself, is called up initially. Everything that then happens is a series of imagined acts, treated as real.

Searching for the essential quality of sequences like this, Csordas notes that in the healing of memories the emergence of the memories themselves is seen as divine revelation, the memories are construed as traumatic and the patient needs to forgive those who caused the trauma, and that in the imaginal performance Jesus enters as the true healer (p. 143). The human healer enters into this sequence by finding a "word of knowledge" through inspiration that leads to the source of trauma. The patient's life is regarded as something unique, therefore access to it is considered divinely caused. Further, the traumatic memory is seen as split off from consciousness, leading to a fragmented sense of the body and the self on the part of the victim. Healers may work with the patient over periods of time and in many sessions before they can identify the trauma and produce the objectified imaginal performance to deal with it. Csordas uses this point (p. 182) to reinforce his argument for incremental efficacy as against miraculous event. From his own evidence we suggest that the relationship between healer and patient *is* also important, even though he himself cautions against seeing the healing efficacy as dependent on this relationship. Ideologically, there seems to be a stress on the patient's own efforts, empowered by God/Jesus. In practice, the healers work with the patients, perhaps over many sessions, they produce the starting images and suggest actions to the patients, and these actions could not be effective without a sense of relationship that entails a mixture of intimacy and control. As Csordas notes (p. 161), in healing, imagery is applied to memory. Our point is that the healer starts this process, *guiding* the patient's imagination, giving it the means to transform itself into a perception of embodied happenings that then acquire an appearance of "inescapable actuality" (p. 163). It is this same guiding power of the healer that brings the patient into "realizing" the original co-presence of Jesus, as a kind of ideal alter ego, and thus entering into the sacred self (p. 164).

Charismatic Catholics recognize vividly the presence of evil, strongly symbolized in the image of demonic possession, and healers practice exorcism in ways that clearly relate to general Catholic tradition. Demons are thought to enter persons who are made vulnerable through trauma, and there is a roster of names for different demons, replacing the medieval roster with abstract terms (Cursing, Depression, Jealousy, etc.; Csordas lists fifty-three root or master spirits/demons, pp. 182–184). Demonic crisis involves losing upright posture and falling to the floor. By contrast "resting in the Spirit," which involves swooning into the arms of catchers and then resting on the floor, is seen as a sign of wellbeing, regularly caused by God. Demonic crisis is thought of as rare, frightening, and caused by Satan. The sacred swoon expresses a blessed release of the self into the divine, marked by intimacy and peace; whereas demonic possession is a violent, disturbing intrusion. Csordas argues strongly that accounts of both need to be seen as accounts of experiences, felt bodily. This argument feeds into his general arguments on healing, since resting in the Spirit is said to make the person relaxed and open to divine healing, so that God may choose that moment to bring a healing about. The calm relaxation conducive to healing is contrasted starkly with the demonic crisis which "epitomizes violence and rage" (p. 261), and is highly active. Its victims may evince flaming eyes and superhuman strength and reject both intimacy with others and control by them (see also Ch. 7 on possession in Haiti). The full exorcism is then required, by which the spirit causing the crisis is "bound" by the name of Jesus and ordered to leave. Csordas further argues that the symptoms displayed in demonic crisis exhibit the traits of major depression, narcissism, and schizophrenia, and are seen as the negatives of the cultural values of spontaneity, intimacy, and control that constitute the relational elements of the sacred self, as well as what we may call its individual elements. Csordas relates these three values further to the practice of speaking in tongues. A neophyte should "step out in faith" (active, individual) but at the same time should "yield to the gift" (passive, relational). Yielding to the gift means responding to God's control over one's life; stepping out in faith means expressing spontaneity; while both are examples of intimate connection with the divine as the "Other" that is also oneself. It is notable that the three values are also realized in bodily action, confirming Csordas's basic proposition that "self processes are orientational processes in which aspects of the world are thematized," so that the self can further be "objectified as a person with a cultural identity"(1997: 64).

Comparisons

Csordas's study both belongs to a general body of literature on forms of religious healing (e.g. McGuire with Kantor 1988; Frank and Frank 1993) and seeks to make a special contribution of its own to the topic of healing, rooted in what he calls "cultural phenomenology." We can define this as the careful depiction of experience as it appears to the experiencing person, a self-account. Such a depiction brings out features that are also found in other analyses of the process of healing in different cultures, as well as some that are not found, or are not developed as fully as they might be. Csordas is not satisfied, for example, with accounts of the healing process that simply depend on the idea of symbolic efficacy (the manipulation of symbols), or that see the key to healing in the healer-patient relationship, or that ascribe healing to the single performance of a ritual act. Rather, his aim is to explore the experience as a temporal process and in full. His two most important contributions are his tying of healing to the remaking of the self and his observation that this remaking is an incremental process.

It is interesting to compare his account with the other two cases we have discussed earlier in this book, (1) curing and healing practices among the Melpa of Papua New Guinea (Chs. 3 and 4), and (2) spiritualist healing in Mexico (Ch. 7).

For the Melpa, as we have learned, sickness conditions may be seen as arising from *popokl* (anger/resentment/frustration). The person who is angry herself/himself becomes sick, but is traditionally supposed to reveal the source of resentment and then those who have done wrong can be asked to make a restitutive payment of wealth to the sick person. The wealth payment then heals the sufferer. In today's Christian version of this way of thinking the sufferer reveals or confesses the anger, but this act of revelation, now seen as a confession, entails that they remove their anger which is distancing them from God. Once they have renounced anger, they will get well.

The Christian version of Melpa thinking, which has become popular only during the 1990s, is clearly very close to the Charismatic Catholic's view that inner healing starts with the revelation of resentment and trauma and with the act of forgiving the wrongdoer. Resentment may not be exactly a sin but it does block the recovery of the sacred self. The feature that is shared by traditional Melpa thought and Charismatic Catholicism in New England is the notion that resentment against others can cause sickness in oneself (the antithesis of witchcraft, which can be thought of as the projection of resentment or malevolence on those causing one to be sick). The exchange-oriented Melpa people felt that the solution was for others to set matters to right by paying compensation: the anger and sickness were directed to wrongdoers, eliciting ideally a restitutive response (or, if this was not forthcoming, retaliatory action where feasible).

The Christian solution is to forgive rather than to fight or to require payment. It places the burden of healing on the self-managing agency of the person, although this cannot work without empowerment by God. Taking the agency back into the person in this sense leads, in the Charismatic case, to the idea of the healing of memories, since traumas can be recalled and then dealt with in the ritual context. It is clear that psychological and psychiatric thinking has considerably influenced the scope of the Charismatics' ideas in this regard. For the Melpa also, *popokl* may be harbored for a long time and lead to chronic sickness, but we do not know of the ritual elicitation of long-standing *popokl* forming, as yet, a part of healing rituals among them. The Melpa idea of the self /person, epitomized in the concept of *noman*, does show some comparability to the idea of the self as orientation and self- process as the work of healing, but the particular emphasis on this view of healing in the Charismatic Catholic movement seems to be attributable to what Csordas calls North American ethnopsychology, with its emphasis on individual responsibility and growth. Perhaps, in the contemporary context of Christianization and modernization, the Melpa idea of "developing a strong *noman*," which has a traditional basis, is itself developing in ways that accommodate it more to the demands of forces similar to those that have shaped North American notions (see Strathern and Stewart 1998).

Csordas's point regarding incremental rather than instantaneous healing is more difficult to discern at work in the Melpa case. There, in the Protestant Pentecostalist churches at any rate, there is indeed a stress on instant, miraculaous healing. But there is perhaps a need, too, for more research on this issue. Csordas notes that his idea can be tested only if there is adequate information on other cases.

Finally, with regard to the Melpa, imagery and imaginal performance are found among them every bit as dramatically as in Csordas's study. For the Melpa, however, much of the work of imagery is done in dream reports and naratives that also reveal self-process in action; whereas Csordas reports that his Charismatics tend to downplay dreams, arguing that these may come from Satan rather than God (1994: 93–5). The Melpa emphasis on dreams is clearly derived from their own traditional culture. Perhaps New England Charismatics see dreams as "pagan"? At least the imaginal performance is found equally in the two cases, however. Our chapter four describes how the Melpa ritual specialist in the past would draw vivid, poetic word pictures of the journeyings of wild spirits, their interactions with the dead kin of the patient, and their own requests to them to depart and leave the sufferer alone: frameworks of depiction that drew the sick person in and enacted the removal of the putative cause of the sickness itself.

The language of these spells is thoroughly imagistic and experiential, depending on the kinds of notions of embodied movement and orientation in space to which Csordas calls attention under his rubric of "phenomenology."

This same point applies strikingly to the Mexican case, as well. Indeed, Finkler's study also shows the applicability of Csordas's idea of "incremental efficacy" to a range of data she surveys. Finkler distinguishes between first-comers, habitual users, and regulars (Finkler 1985: 58–59). In the case of first comers there is little elaboration of imagery employed by healers, although the "haptic technique" of massage is used as a soothing device, the healer seeks inspiration form a guiding spirit, and then pronounces an authoritative diagnosis and treatment, all features also found in the Charismatic universe of healing. With regard to regulars, who join the temple, the following quotation shows the comparability of Finkler's data to those Csordas presents:

"Symbols, of course, are transmitted in various ways, such as during healing and religious rituals to which only regulars are continuously subject. Temple participation thus forms an intrinsic part of the treatment; it exposes participants incessantly to healing and religious rituals.

In Chucha's (a patient's) case the curer linked Chucha's heart-palpitations to crystalline drops falling into an empty glass, the drops symbolizing God's words transmitted during irradiations (services), and Chucha representing the empty glass. Later, Chucha frequently referred to these metaphors" (Finkler 1985: 171–172).

The attendance by regulars at irradiations indicates the incremental effect of the temple rituals *in addition to* the specific healing sessions. The same surely applies in the Charismatic case. The healing image presented to Chucha *transformed* her condition of sickness into an image expressing God's incremental act of filling her with his words. This was also an image of transmuting bodily sickness into spiritual health comparable to the chalice and paten image we gave from Csordas's study. In Chucha's case, she is herself the vessel filled with the word of God; in the Charismatic case the patient filled the chalice with her bitterness (her "sickness") and presented it to Jesus, who transformed it into love (her "healing").

In all of the examples we have reviewed, some aspect, at least, of the *relationship* between healers and patients has proved to be significant, although not solely determinative of the healing process. The Melpa ritual expert derived her/his influence largely from being tied to the patient by kinship, but whether this was so or not the relationship was validated by a payment that also included a *sacrifice* to the dead; the Spiritualist Temple healer in Mexico gains authority through trancing and adopts a commanding tone appropriate to a hierarchical society; the Charismatic healer prays earnestly and "works with" the patient to liberate the patient's sacred self. We stress this point because both Csordas and Finkler argue that the efficacy of healing does not reside greatly "in relationship": our point here is that the overall experience of healing does, nevertheless, involve a culturally appropriate and significant form of relationship-in-action. In Chapter 12 we will look at aspects of communication and relationship again, including biomedicine within our purview. Before doing so, however, we pause to consider the topics of epidemiology (Ch. 10) and fertility and reproduction (Ch. 11).

Chapter 10

Airs, Waters, Places

Environmental medicine is not new. The Hippocratic corpus contains a treatise on the effects exercised by particular environments on the health of their inhabitants. This is the "Airs, Waters, Places" survey, a compendium of observations about places in the Greek world and their effects on health and illness patterns. Epidemiology can rightly trace its lineage back to this ancient, pragmatic, geographically based set of concerns, although in the narrower sense it is focused on the incidence of outbreaks of serious diseases and the statistical patterns of their development over space and time. Epidemiological thinking has also become more complex, as specialists have realized the multiplicity of reasons for the emergence and disappearance of disease patterns, taking in material and topographic factors but also a plethora of social and cultural influences as well as the predominant vectors and characteristics of disease pathogens. Historians and scientists have also often shown the immense effect of epidemics on the course of human history, the defeat of empires not by armies of soldiers but by regiments of disease-bearing organisms, a lesson learned perhaps too well by those states which have developed programs for "germ warfare." Medical anthropology aims to study disease patterns, however, in the context of the everyday lives of people and to see how people interpret them, attempt to combat them, and in any case cope with them.

The Hippocratic treatise on this topic is also closely geared into local practices and thus qualifies as a kind of medical ethnography. Its writer points out that health is affected by the seasons generally, by warm and cold winds and the orientation of the place to these and by the water supply, whether it is marshy and soft or salty and hard. Then there are the local mores: do the people eat or drink heavily or do they eat wisely and drink sparely? (Hippocrates 1978: 148). The writer says that the physician must be his own ethnographer and must make a study of each of these topics. He then proceeds to give some thumbnail typifications of confluent conditions, laying some stress on the influence of winds. In a place where the prevailing winds are warm south-easterlies or south-westerlies, water is plentiful but brackish, and the inhabitants suffer from phlegm that proceeds down from their heads to disturb the inner organs. Their heads are weak and they have a flabby constitution. The women suffer from vaginal discharges and miscarriages, the children are liable to convulsions, and the men suffer from diarrhea, dysentery, ague, and prolonged winter fevers, pustular skin diseases and hemorrhoids, as well as hemiplegia from catarrh. This type of locality (perhaps not unlike the Essex marshlands to be considered later in this chapter) is then contrasted with the case of a district with cold prevailing winds between north-east and north-west. The water is hard, cold, and brackish. The inhabitants are sturdy, lean, liable to constipation, and will suffer from bile more than phlegm, and many have abscesses and pleurisy. The men eat well but drink little. They experience opthalmia, which may become chronic and serious. Their characters tend to be fierce rather than tame. The women suffer from barrenness beause of the hard, cold water, and menstruation is irregular. The children attain puberty at a late age (Hippocrates 1978: 149–151).

It is notable that sketches of this kind touch on all aspects of the human condition including character, and are organized in terms of humoral categories (e.g. phlegm versus bile, and soft versus hard) that putatively exercise a pervasive influence. What we call "the environment" plays a big part in this scheme of thought, but it itself is really assimilated into the humoral scheme of thinking. The treatise proceeds systematically in these terms about a whole range of environmental matters, indicating good and bad features. For example, it declares that the best water comes from high ground, and is sweet and clean, cool in summer but warm in winter because it comes from deep springs. Sick persons should make sure to drink only the best water if it is available, the lightest and most sparkling if the stomach is hard and liable to become inflamed, and the hardest and saltiest if it is soft and full of phlegm. (This belief in the curative powers of pure water much later led to the explosion in the use of natural water sources such as those in Vichy, France, to cure all sorts of ailments and to the popularity of frequenting spas which had a source of water that was said to heal or relieve specific diseases such as that in Baden, Germany. See Maretzki 1989.) In the later part of the treatise the author expands his observations further, arguing for major differences between Asia and Europe and discussing why their people are dissimilar. One of his aims is to delineate how and why people become hard and warlike or soft and peaceloving. His medical ethnography thus easily transforms into political intelligence- gathering in an intriguingly swift move, reminiscent also of Herodotus, the Greek historian, who wrote about the Scythians, Egyptians, and others as this Hippocratic author does. Much later, in the sixteenth and seventeenth centuries in England the idea developed that the place where one was born was the most natural to be in — even though some such places might be unhealthy! (Wear 1995: 166).

This author also identified some of the environmental conditions leading to fevers, including malaria. He linked these to stagnant, stinking water from marshes and lakes, which he thought caused spleens to be enlarged and hard and produced in summertime dysentery and prolonged quartan

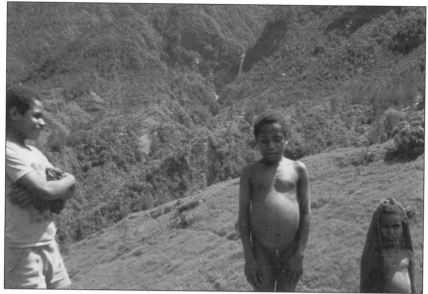

Figure 10–1. Duna landscape. The boy in the middle has a spleen distended from malaria attacks.

fevers. Pregnant and lactating women also suffered from the bad effects of this kind of water. These observations on the relationship between water and fever lead us into considering malaria as a form of epidemic disease.

In this chapter we consider malaria as an example of major epidemic conditions in various parts of the world, looking for some answers to questions concerning the social conditions that produce and are produced by these epidemic diseases. For a part of our materials we go to aspects of European history; for another to more contemporary studies in areas far from Europe such as the Pacific and New Guinea. The past is, indeed, in some ways another country, yet by looking at it we can find parallels with the present if we shift our geographical focus. We choose malaria as an example to illustrate this proposition. Malaria is a serious threat to health and to life itself in many tropical parts of the world today, but it was also a severely debilitating influence in the southeast of England in marshy environments close to the sea, persisting in this regard until the end of the nineteenth century.

Mary J. Dobson, in her book *Contours of Death and Disease in Early Modern England* (1997), analyses the history of malaria in the marshes of Essex, Kent, and Sussex in the seventeenth and eighteenth centuries (compare also Bruce-Chwalt and Zulueta 1980, Ch. 13). It was during this period that the Hippocratic ideas about environmental influences were repopularized and extensive observations were made on minute geographical differences between parishes. Thomas Sydenham, for example, sometimes known as the English Hippocrates, was interested to document "the pestiferous airs and epidemic constitutions of London" (Dobson, p. 19) and his work was very influential. Dobson's own painstaking picture of the 1,185 parishes in the three counties she surveys was built up from consultation of some 1,000 books and their descriptions.

It is remarkable in a study of such detail that the overall epidemiological patterns are outstandingly clear and correspond closely also to the perceptions of observers at the time. The marshy environments less than fifty feet above sea level were places of "bad airs" and "bad waters," pestiferous in the smells that arose from their stagnant pools and with their fogs and mists and clouds of gnats and other insects, and the brackish, sour, dirty waters, unpleasant and noxious to drink. Above that level and in particular above three hundred feet the places were healthy, with fresh air and clean water. As Dobson puts it, "the contours of death and the contours of health were separated by an elevation of little more than 400 or 500 feet," and a distance sometimes of only ten miles (p. 3). Dobson constructs an olfactory map of the southeast of England in which the marshlands uniformly appear marked with a B for "bad air" (p. 14), and a map of the perceptions by vicars of Essex parishes in the eighteenth century in which they chose not to live, the perceptions again coinciding with the extent of the marshlands (p. 296).

As these vicars explained to their bishops, their aversions were based on the experience of illness and the fear of death, primarily from a generic class of conditions all known as the ague. Ague included, but was not limited to, malaria, primarily vivax, which could cause repeated seizures over a period of years before the sufferers succumbed to it. Observers at the time tended to ascribe ague directly to the "marsh vapors" rather than to infection from the bites of mosquitoes. Others declared it arose from the bad drinking water, but this was negated by the fact that in some places the water was clear and pure yet people still fell victims to ague. The term malaria itself, of course, means originally bad air. Other conditions, such as typhus and enteric fever, were also classified as ague, but the fears associated with malaria are distinctive and can be recognized in the symptoms reported by some patients, including enlargement of the spleen and recurrent attacks with intervals of some months in between. In 1807 Arthur Young on a visit to Essex commented on the sallow faces of the inhabitants and swollen bellies of the children (Dobson, p. 315), an observation consistent with malarious conditions.

The presence of malaria is also indicated by the fact that types of ague yielded to large doses of Peruvian bark, containing the alkaloid quinine. The bark was also known as Jesuits' bark, presumably from its use by Jesuit Fathers in South America. One Essex doctor, Robert Talbor, successfully treated King Charles for an ague attack with this bark and was knighted in reward. It was also recognized that the bark could control the ague but not eradicate it from patients. It was expensive and in short supply, and Dobson notes that marsh people tended to rely "more often on herbal cures, charms, opium, and alcohol" (p. 317).

Marsh fever affected village inhabitants regularly (for example Samuel Jeake of Rye who kept a record of his attacks suffered 142 fits between August 1670 and May 1671 and a total of 330 fits altogether between 1667 and 1693, dying at age forty-seven: Dobson pp. 313, 318). Its effects were more severe on visiting strangers. Daniel Defoe told how marshmen took upland brides but regularly lost them through early deaths. Children also suffered more severely than adults (p. 319).

Dobson identifies the *Anopheles atroparvus* mosquito which breeds in estuarine brackish water as the most likely agent for the transmission of malaria, and the type of malaria involved as *vivax* rather than *falciparum*, because the latter requires a temperature of at least twenty degrees Celsius for some three weeks on end for sporogeny. The salt marshes provided the right conditions for the atroparvus vector, and the vivax form of malaria requires a temperature of only sixteen degrees Celsius for sixteen days to complete its sexual cycle, enabling the mosquito to infect humans. Hotter decades were accordingly accompanied by higher mortality levels in marsh parishes, as shown in autumn burial records, though the effects of incubation might be delayed by cold winter weather until the spring following a summer infection. Drought and heat also increased the activities of the atroparvus mosquito, causing it to spread infection more widely.

The impact of malaria in these English marshlands seems to have begun in the sixteenth and seventeenth centuries, possibly as a result of the importation of virulent strains. Even when people did not die directly from attacks of malaria, they were severely debilitated by them and made more susceptible to death from other morbid conditions. Dobson lists (p. 331) more than a dozen such conditions: plague, smallpox, typhoid, dysentery, venereal disease, tuberculosis, brucellosis, typhus, influenza, pneumonia, bronchitis, scarlet fever, whooping cough. Scurvy was also endemic in some low-lying areas, and there was a lack of clean water, leading to cholera and typhoid outbreaks. Dobson notes here that " a mixture of typhoid and malaria infections is a well-known lethal combination in many malarial countries" (p. 336). Finally, malnutrition could both contribute to and be itself exacerbated by malaria, since sufferers would have less appetite.

Obviously, malaria lessened people's capacity to work and increased poverty, and seasonal migrants who entered the marshes were also weakened. Poor women who came in as migrant laborers would suffer pregnancy and childbirth problems and might be less likely to be able to give their infants the protection that breast-feeding provides. Local physicians during the nineteenth century in the Fens noted how infants were sometimes fed by old women with sugar sop, bread fermented with sugar in dirty cups, and poisoned with opium dosages, but it is uncertain whether such conditions also held in preindustrial times.

Ironically, malaria's increasing incidence in the sixteenth century in the marshlands may have been partly the result of lower tidal levels and the fencing of salt-lands for agricultural development. The malaria parasites could have come in with Dutch settlers from the polderlands of Holland. Over time however, through the skills of these same settlers, the marshes were better drained and by the mid-nineteenth century rates of mortality had decreased, although malaria itself remained endemic until the 1920s. A respondent to a medical survey in the 1860s for Maldon in Essex claimed that the ague was sharply reduced in incidence there from its prevalence only twenty years earlier, shown by reduction in spleen enlargements. (Malaria imported by troops in the first World War caused the last epidemic in England, transmitted by the *atroparvus* mosquito *in situ*.) Improved drainage did not by itself eradicate this mosquito, however. Arable farming was improved, and with the introduction of new root crops larger and healthier herds of cows were kept. Possibly mosquitoes came to rely more frequently on cattle for their blood meals than on humans (Dobson, p. 354). People also less often lived alongside their animals. Houses were better ventilated as well. The separation of animals and humans thus protected the human population better. Farmers tried to acquire land for residence in the uplands, combined with marshlands for animal pasture. Interestingly, similar strategies were being advocated at the time in the tropics. (And in the mid twentieth century in the Highlands of Papua New Guinea, plantation owners and government servants invariably attempted to build their houses on raised hills or mounds overlooking the quarters of their laborers, separating themselves both physically and symbolically from the masses.)

In the mid-nineteenth century quinine was first isolated from cinchona (Peruvian) bark, so that its price could accordingly be reduced and its use increased. In some places village people were supplied regularly with quinine powder by their parish parsons. In certain areas resistance to malarial infection may have built up. Malarial infections themselves may have become milder also. Fewer migrants came into the marshlands as these areas were populated through reproductive replacement, and therefore forms of fever such as typhus spread less. Diets improved with the addition of more legumes and fruits, and deep boring for wells brought better supplies of fresh water after 1834 in Essex. Gradually, the use of quinine replaced the use of opium as a treatment for the symptoms of ague, although in some communities old habits continued, at least so long as a pound of opium could be bought for the cost of an ounce of quinine.

Dobson's painstaking study raises many points of interest for comparison with the history of malaria in tropical areas, made sharper by the mild surprise of reading about malaria in southeast England, including London. The past is certainly another country as she shows in fascinating detail. In places such as Papua New Guinea in the Pacific, malaria eradication and treatment programs remain of tremendous importance in the struggle to improve standards of health and survival.

Malaria is in fact a disease that has plagued humans for their entire history. Over a third of the world's population is exposed to risk of malarial infections. In Africa, the form of malaria known as *Plasmodium falciparum* causes at least a million deaths of children each year. Other forms of malaria, *P. vivax*, *P. malariae*, and *P. ovale* are less commonly fatal but are a major cause of global morbidity. Problems in eradicating the disease exist because of the difficulty of ridding areas of mosquitoes and in the spread of resistant strains of the Plasmodium that cannot be treated with chloroquine as they had been previously.

The development of a malarial vaccine has proven to be a particularly challenging problem (see Kwiatkowski and March 1997; Spencer 1994: 150 on Michael Alpers' work). Since malarial conditions exist primarily in countries that are not especially well positioned in the global economy, research funding is not often readily available from internal sources, and external governmental agencies that are situated in countries where malaria is not a great risk factor are less willing to financially support research that does not immediately feed into their own epidemiological profile. Thus, not enough money is available to work on developing a malaria vaccine. In addition to this difficulty there exists the question of how to conduct proper field studies of a vaccine's efficacy. Areas where malaria is endemic often have poor infrastructure for health surveillance which makes the undertaking of a malaria vaccine trial a difficult operation. In some communities over half of the children may be infected with Plasmodium parasites at any time which makes it difficult to evaluate if a fever is attributable to malaria or to various other possible infections, as was the case also in the Essex marshlands.

Archaeological studies show that humans had lived for many generations in the Pacific prior to European exploration into the islands. Written accounts of the European navigators provide some information on the range of infectious agents that existed in the Pacific islands before the nineteenth century. One of these diseases was malaria, mostly of the *Plasmodium vivax* type (Schuurkamp 1992). The disease is thought to have moved into the Pacific islands from Asia through New Guinea and along the Solomon Islands. This might have occurred through the movement of canoes on which the insects or their larvae were carried, or by the movement of small insects in wind currents. Pacific islanders to some extend avoided establishing settlements on coastal strips and swampy areas where mosquitoes breed, but when Europeans established trading posts and missions in the coastal strip areas and native people were attracted to these areas, malaria became a more serious problem (Miles 1997: 19–21).

Generally, the literature on malaria reminds readers of the serious character of the problem of malaria worldwide, its resurgence and the development of chloroquine-resistant strains, and the fact that nevertheless it is in principle controllable by a combination of clinical treatment and public health measures. Desowitz (1991: 123) writes that in a single year "250 million people will get malaria, and at least 2.5 million will die of the infection." Tannes and Vlassof (1997: 523) state that approximately 300–500 million people are infected worldwide, of whom two-three million die each year. As in the case of the English marshlands study, there is an enormous further loss to society in terms of morbidity and inability to work on the part of malaria sufferers. The search for an effective vaccine has not yet been successful. Given this lack of an available overall approach to eradication, local strategies of multiple control remain significant, including the understanding of people's own forms of health-seeking behavior. Tannes and Vlassof stress gendered dimensions of the situation, the high levels of risk for women and children, and the fact that women may have less information than men on treatment options or more information, but less control over family resources. The possibilities for early and effective treatment for women are therefore decreased, they argue (see also Denoon 1989: 112, reporting that in patrilineal communities there may be more concern on the part of fathers to insist on treatment for their sons and heirs than daughters, who are like "bouncing coconuts" that leave on marriage.)

In today's contexts in Papua New Guinea considerations such as Tannes and Vlassof emphasise may apply, but they are overshadowed by larger problems, basically the shortage of medicines in rural Aid Posts. In our own fieldwork in July 1998 among the Duna-speaking people of Aluni in Lake Kopiago, Papua New Guinea, we found that the Aid Post had run out of chloroquine tablets, that the previous supply had in any case been given by a mining company, the Porgera Joint Venture, not by the government, and that people were in general depressed about the lack of rural government services, believing that politicians did not care about the poor rural areas they represented.

Desowitz (1991: 155 ff) recounts some of the alternative ethnotheories advanced as the cause of malaria, mentioning Hippocrates's guess that it was perhaps caused by a dark effluvium rising from the marshes, a speculation that lived in popular thought in the Essex marshes in the eighteenth century, as we have seen. A spraying campaign in the Philippines in 1996 collapsed because the local people thought malaria was caused by a combination of pollution in water and fatigue. The Roman writer

Marcus Varro thought it was caused by unseen animals that infest the air and water in swamps (c. 50 BC). Carolus Linnaeus wrote his Doctor of Medicine dissertation in 1735 on malaria, and starting from Hippocrates' observations about the dark color of the spleen in patients with swamp fever which Hippocrates attributed to black bile, he suggested instead it was from suspended clay particles in drinking water that occluded the body's organs and caused the fever. The microscope had been invented as early as 1674 but it was not until 1870 that Louis Pasteur finally established microbes as causative agents of specific diseases. The protozoan parasite that causes malaria had been adequately observed and described by 1895, and gradually epidemiologists came to replace the Hippocratean miasma theory of its transmission with a theory of mosquito-borne transmission. A little ironically, the evidence for this came at least partly from reports that natives in parts of Africa and Asia said the disease was caused by mosquito bites. The first definitive discovery that the female anopheles mosquito transfers the sporozoite forms of the parasite through its salivary glands by biting in order to obtain a blood meal was made by a British scientist Robert Ross in 1898 in Calcutta, followed closely by the Italian Giovanni Grassi in 1899. The discovery clearly pointed to the importance of curtailing the lifecycles of the mosquitoes and of avoiding mosquito bites, thus ushering into the twentieth century the possibility of public health programs along these lines.

It is interesting to note here that local peoples everywhere have had an accurate *practical* knowledge of how to avoid getting malarial fevers. The Essex marshlanders knew that their places were unhealthy but had nowhere else to go. In New Guinea populations that live in low-lying swampy areas filled with mosquitoes attempt to avoid getting bitten by these by sleeping inside baskets or by situating their houses on breezy knolls. Mountainside Duna dwellers of the Southern Highlands Province in PNG, living in cooler higher-altitude sites where mosquitoes are blown away by wind and water runs away quickly in runnels, especially in limestone country, openly declare that the low altitude areas near to the Strickland River Gorge are unhealthy by comparison and that people who live there get sick and die more quickly. They trace the origins of witchcraft practices to these low-lying areas and see witches as the descendants,mostly female, of the original groups that emanated from the Strickland and migrated uphill. If such people originally brought with them both malarial parasites and a greater acquired resistance to them they might well have been the agents of fatal sickness among those kinsfolk into whose places they came, thus possibly increasing the likelihood that they might be identified as witches, since their arrival brought death to others and not to themselves. This is just a speculation, in line with earlier speculations by Inge Riebe on the Kalam people (Riebe 1987), but it underlines the point that local forms of knowledge about disease patterns usually encode an accurate perception of the environment at one level, even if they invoke mystical concepts such as witchcraft at another level. Also, the origin of witchcraft in the Duna area (which is often stated as the cause of deaths from epidemics) is said to be from a hole in the earth at the Strickland from which a male cannibalistic spirit (*tama*) came forth and was prepared to kill and eat a female victim but decided to take her as a sexual partner instead, thereby transferring his powers of witchcraft to her and thence to her offspring.

Witchcraft-induced diseases are often seen as arising from watering holes such as those found in swampy areas where mosquitoes breed. We can therefore see a connection arising in people's minds between ecological conditions and disease, mediated by ideas such as that of witchcraft which stand in the place of ethnotheories of microbes or parasites.

Malaria certainly continues to be a serious problem in tropical countries such as Papua New Guinea. There is a fairly long history of public health efforts to deal with it, linked also to North Queensland, where Melanesian laborers were recruited to work in sugarcane plantations up until 1904. Outbreaks of malaria in Queensland and the Northern Territory of Australia were sometimes a result of importations from New Guinea by Australian miners who worked in both places. The Australian Institute of Tropical Medicine was set up partly to handle research into malaria and was the first institute of medical research in Australia, opened in Townsville in January 1910 (Spencer 1994: 15). This was just four years after Australia had taken over from Britain colonial responsibility for Papua, the southern half of what in 1975 became the nation of Papua New Guinea. The Institute was also concerned with filariasis and with dengue fever. Missionary organizations such as the Anglican Church in Papua were also involved, since many of their workers died of malaria while at work in the field. The Institute became a part of the Federal Department of Health in 1921, which established a branch laboratory in Rabaul off the northern coast of New Guinea. Dr. Raphael West Cilento was for some time both Director of the Institute at Townsville and Director of Health and Quarantine in New Guinea. Cilento summed up available knowledge about malaria in New Guinea and Papua in the 1920s, and pointed out that mosquito extermination should always be undertaken with careful consideration of the local ecology of the mosquitoes themselves—an enterprise which we may add would depend much on the knowledge of local people themselves.

As the historian Donald Denoon has pointed out, we need to distinguish between concern for the white colonial population and concern for the health of indigenous people (Denoon 1989: 22). The best approaches to "tropical medicine," such as those of Sir William MacGregor, the energetic Lieutenant-Governor of British New Guinea (later Papua) from 1888–1898, surely combined a legitimate interest in both of these domains of health. MacGregor, in particular, advocated environmental medicine as the means to ensure the health of all categories of people, for example by securing the purity of the water supply (quoted in Denoon 1989: 22).

World War II with its action against Japanese forces in New Guinea brought renewed interest and concern over malaria, fostered by Dr. John Gunther who was working as a malariologist for the RAAF there in wartime and in 1946 was appointed Director of Public Health in Papua and New Guinea. Gunther stressed the disruptive and debilitating effects of malaria on the local populations, including those employed on work at plantations in coastal areas. In one of his writings he argued "control malaria and add 15% to the individual laborer; control malaria and reduce the potential need for labor by 25%; control malaria and therefore save hundreds of thousands of pounds." He also pointed out that malaria control would improve the aptitude of students in educational institutions (Spencer 1994: 74). Both DDT spraying and oiling of larval ponds had been used to assist in such control programs, though Gunther was skeptical about the former as applied to houses since female mosquitoes might not rest long enough inside houses to receive a lethal dose. He gave priority to larval control. Such arguments again might depend on local knowledge of mosquito behavioral patterns.

Another scientist, Stanley Christian, carried out surveys in the recently opened-up Highlands areas, showing malaria was endemic above 1,650 meters in the Wahgi and Chimbu areas though absent eastwards in the Goroka Valley. Gambusia affinis fish which eat mosquito larvae were brought to the Highlands as a part of the control effort. Gunther also set up the Native Medical Orderly training program in 1947. Laws were made to administer malaria protection to Highlanders recruited to work on the coast, and in the Highlands itself large drainage schemes were undertaken, for example at Minj and Banz, which helped to pave the way for coffee and tea plantations to be set up.Gunther also set up a Malaria Control School at Minj in 1954, to be attended by field officers stationed throughout the country. A malariologist, Dr. Wallace Peters, was appointed in 1956 and began a series of epidemiological studies. Peters' work included attention to rates of human splenomegaly and also to vector patterns of adult female mosquitoes in differing locations. He recognized that malaria would spread in the Highlands with the development of roads and advocated residual DDT spraying up to about 1,800 meters with the aim of malaria eradication rather than simply control. Gunther hoped that villagers would voluntarily carry out the spraying, but in fact they usually asked to be paid for work of this kind. Peters' surveys also showed that *Plasmodium vivax* was the dominant form of infection, the more dangerous *Plasmodium fal-*

ciparum not exceeding 30%–40% (although later studies tend to show that *falciparum*, including chloroquine-resistant types, is on the increase today). Dr. Roy Scragg, appointed Director of Public Health in Papua New Guinea in succession to Gunther in 1957, stressed in 1959 that the malaria problem was tied in with issues medical anthropologists will recognize: education, development, housing, land use, and what he called "the fundamental ignorance of the indigenous people of the real basis of the diseases that affect them" (quoted in Spencer 1994: 105).

Here we may comment that another approach would be to document what people do to avoid being bitten by mosquitoes regardless of whether they think they cause malaria—i.e. by the use of smoke, oil or ashes on the skin, house-siting, draining and trenching, etc. Further, their symbiotic patterns with animals such as dogs and pigs should be studied for the likely effect on biting patterns. We are reminded here of Dobson's observation from Essex of smallholders who arranged pigstyes around their houses to encourage the mosquitoes to bite the pigs before reaching the humans (Dobson 1997: 354). In the Highlands pigs have often been stalled at night in women's houses for safekeeping and feeding. How would that affect the biting patterns of mosquitoes? Fires are also traditionally made in all houses, which would discourage mosquitoes. These patterns have been modified by cultural changes, in which pigs are kept separately from people and houses are sometimes made without fires in imitation of European patterns.

One final topic from Spencer's study is interesting. She mentions work on TSS, Tropical Splenomegaly Syndrome, which showed that in the Maprik area of New Guinea in 1971 malaria control had achieved little reduction of cases of grossly enlarged spleens leading to mortality. The transition from simple malarious splenomegaly to TSS seems to have occurred between six and twenty years of age in patients, but antimalarial drugs were effective in reducing spleen size in 73% of subjects treated (Spencer 1994: 137)

This is interesting in terms of our points made above about local knowledge and perceptions. In the Duna area in mid-1998 people frequently came to us complaining of "spleen" (a term used also earlier in 1991). It was this rather than fever that they commented on as the evidence of their sickness. It may be that there was a prior existing indigenous interest in the spleen (*hayeni* in the local language) since pigs' spleens were used in certain rituals. Or it may simply be that this was how the people had been educated into malaria awareness. In any case their concern was marked, and perhaps justifiably if they had a tendency to develop TSS as was found in the Maprik study.

1998 was a crucial year to be studying issues of epidemics in Papua New Guinea since 1997–98 saw the long, drawn-out debilitating effects of the severe El Niño induced drought there, followed by rains and a spread of renewed epidemic disease outbreaks, including malaria. Dr. Michael Bourke, a Human Geographer at the Australian National University employed on health surveys in Papua New Guinea during the drought, reported that there was widespread evidence for malaria epidemics during this period, perhaps associated with people spending more time foraging in the bush (ASAO Net March 23, 1998). This fact reminds us that malaria control has not approached malaria eradication yet in most parts of Papua New Guinea, and malaria always has the ability to return in times of recurrent stress, a fact that is recognised as being true for other major epidemic conditions such as tuberculosis.

With malaria there is also the problem of the loss of resistance to the disease that accompanies the use of prophylactic doses of drugs in contexts of holoendemic prevalence of the condition, and correlatively the development of resistance to the drugs by mutant forms of the disease.

Our own experience is that Papua New Guinea villagers quickly learn to seek the help of introduced medicines such as chloroquine tablets for malaria, even if they respond more slowly to public health injunctions about environmental management. Their recent response to the onset of AIDS in their communities indicates their awareness of how much worse things are when there are as yet no known medicines. In fact by 1976 it was accepted that available insecticides and drugs could not stop transmission of malaria, and this led to a change in direction of malaria research with an intensification of interinstitutional effort on all fronts, including drugs, vaccines, diagnosis, and vector control.

In Papua New Guinea this research has been directed from the Institute of Medical Reserach in Goroka by Dr. Michael Alpers since 1979, and the complex search for a vaccine has continued as a part of the program. Human malaria vaccine trials were proposed to be commenced by the end of 1991, but as of 1998 no fully acceptable vaccine had been developed for regular immunological use that could prevent the condition, which became so devastatingly prevalent in earlier decades in African countries as well as in America and Europe.

We do not deal with AIDS as such here, although much anthropological research has been dedicated to it especially in the context of applied anthropology and ethnic studies in the USA, but we do wish to draw attention to early phases of narrative construction about it in our field areas in Papua New Guinea since such accounts are not so commonly found in the literature. (For an explanation of narratives about immunity and the immune system in the U.S.A. "from the days of Polio to the Age of AIDS," see Martin 1994).

In the Hagen area of Papua New Guinea AIDS was not discussed with us as a disease that the people had an awareness of until mid-1998 when everyone had suddenly become cognizant of the disease through both the newspapers and the local churches. Moreover, a specific narrative had developed, widely shared, that a famous rugby player from one of the Hagen tribes had gone overseas and there had intercourse in a hotel room with a woman who announced she was attracted to him. She left him a note saying "Welcome to the world of AIDS" and departed before he woke. On his return home, he underwent a test and was found HIV-positive.

In this narrative it was clear that the rugby player had been tricked into having sex with the woman who was carrying the HIV virus, that the woman (who was not a New Guinean) had plotted to transmit the disease to this man knowing that she was infected, and that the man would spread the disease to others upon his return to New Guinea. Interestingly the man is said to have been told by the woman that she had AIDS and yet he is said to have continued to have sexual relations both with his wives and with other women. Thus, both the woman who first infected the man is seen as being outside of the moral restraints that would govern conduct between people and the man is seen as being outside of these moral restraints after becoming infected. This in turn is given as the reason for his affliction with AIDS.

In our Hagen field area the people reported being told in the churches not to have extramarital sexual relations and not to marry a person until an HIV blood test had been conducted. All of our informants said that they had been told that the disease AIDS was transmitted through sexual intercourse but most people also thought that the disease could be transmitted through mosquito and louse bites. Some thought that sharing drinking cups and eating utensils could also spread the disease. No one was prepared to name any of those who were infected with the virus but all claimed to know which families had infected persons in them. It was declared that men die in 4–5 years after contracting the disease while women, who are weaker, die after 2–3 years. Generalizing from the case of the rugby player, people declared also that it was men with money who travelled abroad that brought the disease back and infected young girls with it through giving them money for sex.

In a part of the Duna area in the Southern Highlands Province AIDS was said to have arisen just in 1998. No persons who had the disease were named but one woman from a distant parish was reported to have died from it. The condition was said to have come from the "islands" into New Guinea.

We may compare these incipient forms of narrative in Papua New Guinea with the more established ones found by the anthropologist Brad Weiss among the Haya people during 1988–90 in Tanzania, East Africa, where AIDS appears to have become prevalent over a period of years (Weiss 1992). Weiss examines the phenomenon of "plastic teeth" and their extraction, said by the Haya to be a recent pathological intrusion into their lives. Small children are declared to grow plastic teeth instead of normal ones, and these must be removed because they cause diarrhea, vomiting, fever, and wasting. The growth of teeth in children is linked by the Haya to proper forms of developmental patterns and kinship relations, and further to ideas of agency, naming, and the capacity for speech. In other words, the mouth and its teeth are a microcosm of the Haya social world, so that anomalous events in the mouth may reasonably be connected to anomalous circumstances in the Haya lived world. Plastic is seen as a foreign substance that can assume various forms and is therefore a quintessential example of the commodity and the process of commoditization that affects the Haya. A plastic tooth supplanting a real one shows a perversion of growth and a threat to proper biological and social reproduction. As a perceived recent epidemic from outside, the plastic teeth syndrome reflects, Weiss suggests, the Haya's weak position in a world where they sell coffee for declining prices, experience land fragmentation, and suffer from arbitrary currency devaluations of their money. He goes on to point out that these ideas about plastic teeth run parallel to ideas about AIDS. "Like plastic teeth, AIDS is said to have originated in Uganda and to have come to Kagera (among the Haya) through the sexual contacts of rich Haya businessmen." Furthermore, both plastic teeth and AIDS are said to cause wasting of the body, and an inability to make proper use in the body of food ingested through the mouth (the Haya make classic connections between eating and sexuality also). Contrasting AIDS and plastic teeth, however, one man said that plastic teeth are a kind of children's "Slim" (AIDS) but there are doctors who can cure it, whereas adults have no medicine for AIDS, and they simply die (Weiss 1992: 546).

Although the narratives in Papua New Guinea have not yet reached the symbolic complexity of the Haya case, the basic standpoint is the same. AIDS, seen as a product of the deleterious aspects of globalization, has also become a signifier of corruption linking together the illicit flow of sexual behavior in a fragmenting world.

Chapter 11

Fertility

Concerns over fertility are one of the major underlying factors in many ritual practices around the world, and much time and energy as well as resources are funnelled into activities to ensure that fertility is retained within a population. Many of the ritual practices that deal with removing sickness in general from a community, such as those discussed earlier (Chapters 3, 4, 5) for the Hagen and Duna areas of Papua New Guinea, are also aimed at increasing fertility.

Fertility is frequently envisioned in terms of the female and male fluids that feed into conception. McGilvray's study of sexual power and fertility in Sri Lanka has shown that in the Batticaloa region people have a notion of two semens: one male and the other female (1994). Female semen is said to be found in the uterus and is thought to be a derivative of blood. Fertilization take place when these two substances mix and fetal development is said to occur directly by maternal blood nourishing the child through its fontanelle at the top of its head. The cessation of menstruation during pregnancy is thought to occur because of the diversion of blood needed to nourish the developing fetus.

In Batticaloa, when a woman is unable to become pregnant she frequently seeks treatment in the domain of traditional medicine. This may require the use of a mixture of herbal compounds, prescribed in accordance with instructions encoded in medical songs that are mnemonic devices and are recited from beginning to end. The various ingredients used in treating infertility are drawn from the traditional Ayurvedic pharmacopoeia and are available for purchase in local herbal stores. The treatments are aimed at restoring a humoral balance. There is also the notion that infertility can be caused by malevolent spirits acting on their own or as agents sent through sorcery. To counter this a woman may recite *mantra* or ask a Hindu deity or Muslim saint for assistance in becoming pregnant.

Fertility can be affected by a host of diseases some of which reduce fecundability, causing sterility (McFalls and McFalls 1984). Sexually transmitted diseases can cause infertility through scarring of fallopian tubes after an infection has occurred. Gonorrhea is a common cause of tubal occlusion, ectopic pregnancy, persistent lower abdominal pain, and infertility in women.

The problem of infertility is dealt with in a variety of ways in different cultural contexts. Among the Aowin people of southwest Ghana, different

153

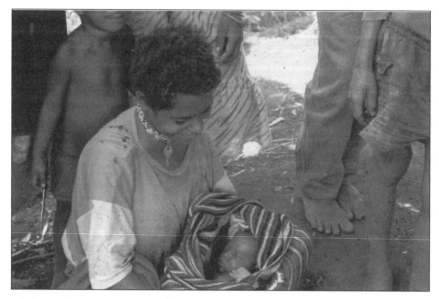

Figure 11–1. Mother with young infant in netbag (Duna).

types of healers are available to help resolve this condition: spirit mediums who are female and herbalists who are male (in the past men used to also act as spirit mediums but have ceased to do so) provide two avenues of treatment that can be sought in addition to the government hospital, Muslim healers and Christian healers. Aowin rarely depend on just a single healer, changing practitioners if they do not meet with success after being treated by their first choice (Ebin 1994: 131–134).

Fertility is an index of the relationships of an Aowin with the spirit world and is tied to the general state of the cosmos. Sterile men and women are never fully accepted as members of the society and barren women may be suspected of being witches. Women in Aowin are credited with special powers that allow them to bear children. It is believed that the gods are angry with a woman if she is infertile. For the spirit medium, the patient's social relationships are the central issue of treatment. Troubled relations with the spirit world can bring misfortune such as infertility to a family. In V. Ebin's study of women who sought treatment from spirit mediums several diagnoses and treatments were offered. (1) Some women were told that they were witches. (2) Others were told that they had offended the gods by not observing traditional purification practices and neglecting to provide the appropriate offerings to them, and thus had acquired pollution, *efeya*, which prevented conception. (3) Another group of women were advised that they could not conceive because they had *efeya* which had come

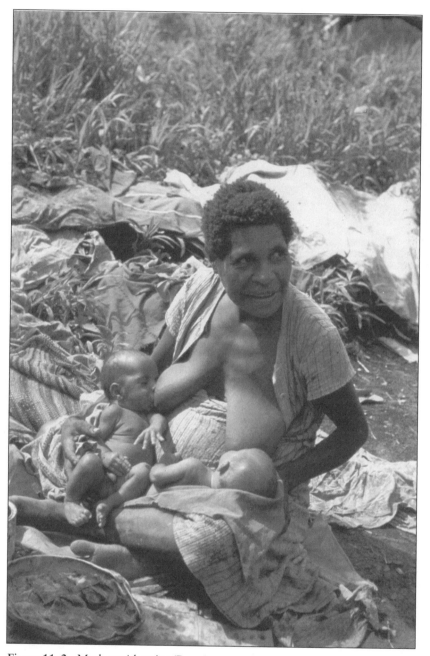

Figure 11–2. Mother with twins (Duna).

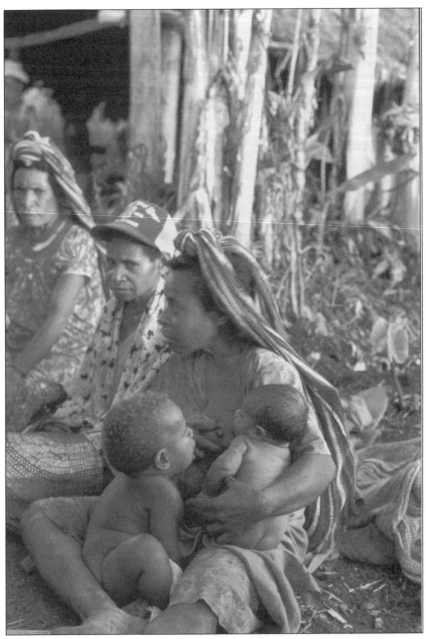

Figure 11–3. Mother with two infants, both dependent on her milk (Duna).

from unreconciled personal relationships such as quarrels with husbands or cowives. (4) Other women were said to be infertile because their behavior had generated a tension within the matrilineal group, which is considered a serious offense that creates a state called *monzue* and can threaten the wellbeing of the individual as well as the entire community.

For these categories, the spirit medium suggested treatments of (1) purification, (2) therapeutic remedies, and (3) reconciling social relations. Purification requires that the woman bathe in the river and give a modest offering to the gods such as eggs or a hen. After this the medium paints the woman with clay and leads the woman back to the town. When the woman's offense has been great enough to endanger the safety of the entire town the woman may need to spend weeks with the spirit medium in the forest at the medium's shrine undergoing daily remedies valued for their purification properties such as eating specified foods and cleaning the body daily. At the end of her purification period, her kinsfolk go to the medium's shrine to participate in the offering of a sheep to the gods, who are then requested to remove the *monzue* pollution. A second form of treatment available to these women is therapeutic. Here the spirit medium administers various plant remedies. Thirdly, the spirit medium recommends reconciling disturbed social relations (Ebin 1994: 135–142).

In addition to the spirit medium's set of diagnoses and treatments patients may seek the help of male herbalists who listen to the patients' physical complaints and attempt to determine what might be causing the infertility. The herbalist does not consider difficulties in personal relationships as affecting the woman's health and does not attempt to modify her behavior in order to effect a cure. His treatments are solely aimed at what might be the anatomical or physiological difficulty in the woman's body that leads to her infertility.

In the Hagen, Pangia, and Duna areas of Papua New Guinea, concerns over infertility found their expression in a number of fertility rituals such as the Amb Kor (Female Spirit) cult in Hagen that was held periodically to ensure that women would bear children and that the fertility of the ground as well as of the livestock (pigs) would continue. If these ritual practices were carried out properly the Amb Kor would place part of her fertility powers in the cult stones that the ritual performers had gathered to honor her. These stones would be surrounded by cool ferns and anointed with pork fat (*kng kopong*, symbolizing semen) and red ochre (*ui kela*, symbolizing blood) and then be buried in the local soil of the group at the conclusion of the cult ritual performance (Strathern and Stewart 1998; Stewart 1998).

The Amb Kor is just one example of a series of Female Spirits found in the Highlands of New Guinea who were looked to as sources of fertility (Stewart and Strathern 1998). In Pangia the local Female Spirit was called the Aroa Ipono while in Duna she was known as the Payame Ima. In addition to these Female Spirit cults other fertility rituals were practised which

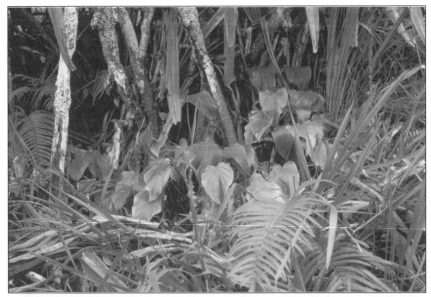

Figure 11–4. (1991) *Palena*, plants for magically increasing the growth of pigs and people, near to Aluni (Duna).

involved the presentation of bodily substances to spirits living within the ground. In the Duna area *hambua hatya* was a ritual that took place along an extended trackway between the parish of Yokona, near to the Strickland river and Lake Kopiago, and a sacred site located far to the south in the territory of the Huli people called Kelokili. The ritual putatively involved human sacrifice and dismemberment. Parts of a victim's body were said to have been buried at specific cult spots; some of these body parts were said to have been reserved for the cannibal spirit Hambua who was thought to abide in a hole at Kelokili (P. J. Stewart 1998). Another fertility ritual complex from the Duna area that involved the movement of body parts along a trackway between the Strickland river and the Kelokili was the *kirao hatya*. In this ritual menstrual blood was collected from a virgin of a particular descent group and was carried along the trackway until reaching Kelokili where it was placed into a hole in the earth (A. Strathern and P. J. Stewart 1998). The woman who donated her menstrual blood was expected to remain a virgin for the rest of her life in a manner reminiscent of the vestal virgins in ancient Rome. In these rituals the idea was to bring fertility to humans and animals and renew the fertility of the ground so that crops would grow well and foods would be plentiful.

Fertility rituals were historically imported into the Hagen and Pangia areas with a set of ideas about how gender relations should be structured. In both Pangia and Hagen the Female Spirit cults were a means of not just

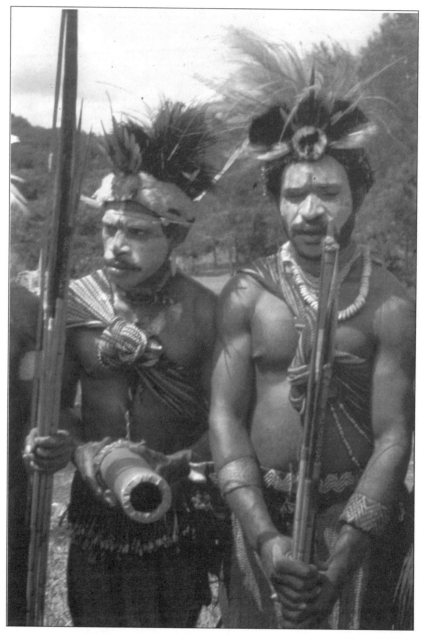

Figure 11–5. Duna youths decorated for dancing. Their attire partially resembles that of boys who used to emerge from the *palena* house where they were ritually "grown" by a cult expert.

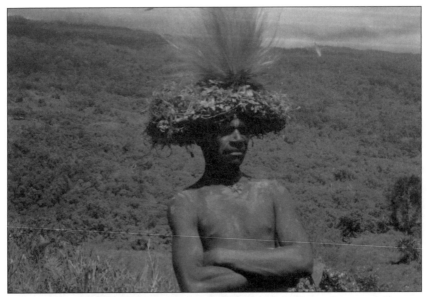

Figure 11–6. A youth of the age that in the past was secluded in the growth house. His wig is built from human hair and vines.

bringing fertility but also of providing protection to men against the potentially lethal powers of menstrual blood. It was thought that menstrual blood could produce sickness and even death in a man if taken in through the penis or the mouth by ingestion of contaminated food. Thus, women were segregated off from men into special menstrual huts where they would cook their own food and would not prepare food for their spouse or male relations during their cycle of menstrual flow. Interestingly, in Pangia it was thought that if menstrual blood did come into a man it could potentially produce an ectopic pregnancy which would eventuate in death because of the lack of a uterus and vagina to expel the fetus from the body (Stewart and Strathern 1998). (All of these ritual practices have ceased in these areas now that the people are Christians.)

In Hagen when a woman does become pregnant conception is described as an event that initially involves the mixing of the sexual *kopong* (grease) of the female (vaginal fluids) and that of the male (semen) as a first step. This is followed by the male *kopong* surrounding the *mema* (blood) of the female to produce a fetal packet like an egg (*köi mukl*), described as *kum ronom*, "it wraps." This packet will become a child if nurtured in the womb (Strathern and Stewart 1998b). This embodied sequence of actions is paralleled by the stone-burying rituals at the conclusion of the Female Spirit cult, detailed above.

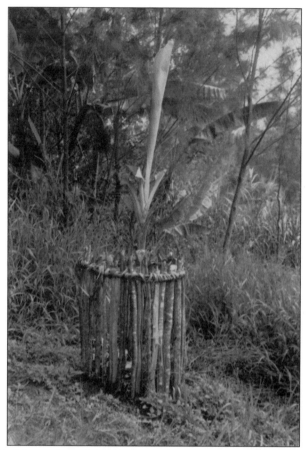

Figure 11–7. Hagen. A special enclosure built to contain the afterbirth and umbilical cord of a child in order to "root" the child in the land. A banana shoot grows in the enclosure, marking powers of growth and renewal (Kawelka Kundmbo).

Although it has been stated by some writers that people in the Hagen area of Papua New Guinea do not have an idea of the fetus being nurtured in utero, this does not correlate with interviews that we conducted during 1997–98 with both men and women of various age groups in the Hagen area. Hageners realize that during pregnancy the child grows and becomes bigger and that special foods must be eaten to ensure the health of the growing child. It is clear from the narrative given below that both the *kopong* (grease) and the *mema* (blood) of the female sustains and nurtures the developing child in utero. The category of *kopong* includes the nurturant quality of foods that are especially eaten during pregnancy such as greens, other juicy vegetable foods, and pork fat. Also, red-colored

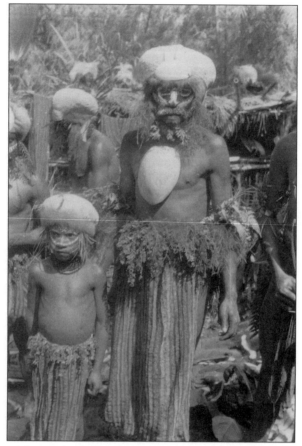

Figure 11–8. (1973) A dancer for the Female Spirit cult in Hagen with his small son (his "banana shoot") (Kawelka Kundmbo).

foods are thought to help to replenish the blood and are eaten at this time. Male *kopong* (semen) is thought to be deleterious during pregnancy and during the period of breast feeding since it is believed to "spoil" breast milk, hence there is a taboo on intercourse during pregnancy and during the post-partum breast feeding years (see chapter three for more details on Melpa humoral ideas).

One of our Hagen informants (Mr. Ru-Kundil), who is a local specialist on traditional knowledge, described the process of growth that occurs during gestation in utero as follows:

"It was previously thought [before health care workers told Hageners otherwise] that a woman had two cords inside of herself that fed into the growing child. One cord was a path for the woman's blood to flow into the

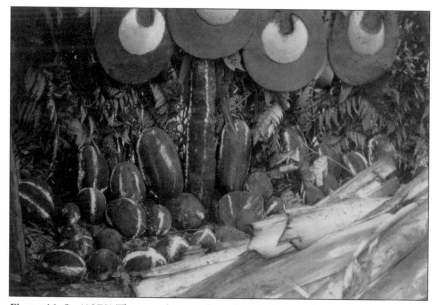

Figure 11–9. (1970) The sacred stones for a Female Spirit cult performance. Banana stocks cover an earth oven in front of them, where pork is steaming. Pearl shells on backings are suspended above them.

child (the umbilicus) and the other went to her breast and carried her milk to the growing child."

While not all Hageners described this two-cord nurturance system, all spoke of the mother's blood carrying growth-sustaining fluids derived from the foods that the mother ate during her pregnancy. The mother is therefore definitely seen as more than just a vessel or container for the child.

Duna ideas of conception involve the mixing together of male "water" and female blood but not grease. This fits with their humoral system which does not rely on grease as the Melpa one does but is based on ideas of blood and water, where water takes the place of grease (see Ch. 3). The Duna also believe that the child grows in utero through the foods that the mother eats. These are thought to replenish/fortify her blood which then enters the growing fetus through the umbilical cord.

In both the Hagen and Duna areas infertility is a highly undesirable state for a woman and can be a cause for a husband to take another wife (polygamy is legal in Papua New Guinea although moves are afoot to pass legislation to outlaw the practice) and/or send the infertile wife back to her kinsfolk.

Infertility is a concern for people globally. In the United States, many couples who experience infertility increasingly seek to remedy the problem

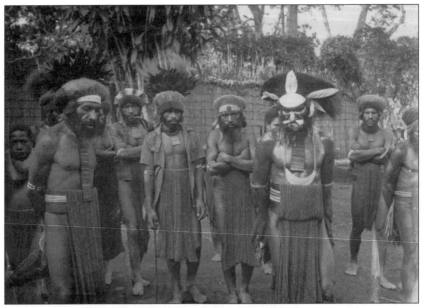

Figure 11–10. (1969) Kope tribesmen preparing for a Female Spirit performance make a serious count of pig stakes in front of the cult enclosure. Pigs attached to these stakes will be given away prior to the cult performance to strengthen the group's ties with its allies.

through medical procedures. Literature available on infertility suggests that failure to conceive after one year of unprotected intercourse indicates that a fertility problem may exist. Diagnosis and treatment is an expensive endeavor. A basic postcoital test may cost several hundred dollars. Ovulation inducing drugs are costly as well, which limits the possibility for everyone to seek this sort of treatment. There can also be dangerous side-effects such as the inducement of premature menapause or stimulation of multiple ovulation leading to multiple births. When in vitro fertilization methods are used a woman may undergo multiple egg retrieval procedures. These procedure can produce discomfort and require the woman to monitor her ovulatory cycle so as to be at the clinic at the correct time to maximize the likelihood of extracting healthy, ripe eggs that will be receptive to sperm penetration in vitro.

Once an embyro has been cultured in the laboratory it next needs to be implanted into a female uterus so that it can attach itself onto the uterine wall and begin development in the normal physiological way. For a number of technical reasons, embryo transfers do not always "take" (i.e., lead to pregnancy) and thus the patient may need to receive repeated embryo transfers over time in order to effect a single pregnancy.

The infertility business is a multibillion dollar industry in the U.S. and has raised a plethora of ethical, medical, and legal concerns. Issues of identity and parental rights are often difficult to assess in situations where donor sperm and/or donor eggs are used to create embryos that will subsequently be implanted into the genetic mother or a surrogate mother (referred to as a "gestational carrier") in order for gestation to be completed.

In addition to the problems that arise out of the new reproductive technology that we have discussed so far in this section issues of ambiguous kinship ties can arise which require legal expertise to help resolve. For example, a case reported in the New England Journal of Medicine describes a particularly complex set of relationships from which a child was brought into being, but in a context that resulted in a judge declaring that the child was parentless even though his creation involved at least five adults (Annas 1998). The case involved a couple who opted to have a child using in vitro fertilization methods. In this case both the eggs and sperm were donated for the procedure. The viable embryo that was produced from these donated gametes was implanted into a genetically unrelated woman who carried the pregnancy to term for the couple. Although the couple commissioned the creation of this child intending to rear it as their own, before the birth occurred the two separated and the nongenetic "father-to-be" of the child wanted nothing to do with it. The legal case that followed declaring the child parentless was overturned in appeals court in California with the decision stating that, "a husband and wife should be deemed the lawful parents of a child after a surrogate bears a biologically unrelated child on their behalf…since in each instance a child is procreated because a medical procedure was initiated and consented to by intended parents" (Annas 1998 citing Buzzanca v. Buzzanca 1998).

Another example involved a woman living in New York who had undergone five egg-retrieval procedures and nine embryo transfers, none resulting in a live birth. The woman and her husband decided to seek a surrogate mother to assist them. This required that they sign consent forms allowing the embryos to be produced and the procedure to take place. An addendum to one of the forms stated that if they (the genetic parents) "no longer wish to initiate a pregnancy or are unable to make a decision regarding the disposition of our stored, frozen pre-zygotes…they may be disposed of by the in vitro fertilization program" (Annas 1998). The couple were unsuccessful in creating a child and subsequently divorced. The woman sought to obtain custody of the frozen embryos for her own use but her ex-husband opposed this. Initially a trial court granted custody of the embryos to the woman but the decision was overturned by higher courts and the embryos were not retained (Annas 1998).

Both of these examples show how reproductive technology involves courts as well as clinics. Although individual states within the U.S. have jurisdiction over defining parenthood and child custody, issues arising out of assisted reproductive technology pose a new set of questions that are often difficult to reach decisions on, such as the type of records that should be kept on egg and sperm donations; the rights of children created by these procedures to know the identities of their genetic and gestational parents and their rights to potentially make legal and/or psychological demands of them; and the percentage of "motherhood" that should be afforded gestational and genetic mothers.

The same question of the definition of motherhood and the rights pertaining to it came up crucially in 1986 in the state of New Jersey when Mary Beth Whitehead acted as surrogate mother of a child for the married couple William and Elizabeth Stern under a contract drawn up by the Infertility Center of New York. In this instance Mr. Stern's sperm was inseminated into Mrs. Whitehead to fertilize her egg, and as part of the contract she specifically agreed to give up her maternal rights to Mr. Stern. However, in giving birth to the child Mary Whitehead was overcome by feelings of guilt and by the idea that she was really selling her child "like a slave" (i.e. as a transitional object without automatic rights of kinship) (Fox 1997: 57). She and her husband resisted the attempts of the Sterns to claim the child, who became known as "Baby M," and were subjected to police hunts and arrests until the matter was brought again to court and the rights of the *genitor*, Mr. Stern, were upheld against the *genetrix* rights of Mrs. Whitehead. Robin Fox, who discusses the case, actually became involved in it as a "friend of the court" (*amicus curiae*), pointing out the strength of mother-child bonding in mammalian populations, but to no avail. The law of contract was upheld against the rights of motherhood. Fox also points out that the reason why there was such a struggle and the courts found the matter hard to decide was that there was no applicable precedent in law, and the actual situation scrambled the applicability of existing law. This points up the fact that biotechnology can sometimes lead to very painful and wrenching emotional and legal conflicts, while in other circumstances it helps people to fulfill their dreams. It is in this regard a Pandora's box that, once opened, can never be closed. The imaginations of people can also act as a source of actual problems through their fantasized pictures of what is possible, as we shall see next.

Severed Fingers and Biotechnology
The Synecdochal Person

Our examples in this chapter, taken from indigenous societies of New Guinea and from the United States, indicate the immense value placed on fertility by populations throughout the world. Highlanders of New Guinea developed elaborate ritual practices, linking human fertility with the reproduction of the cosmos, which entailed the slaughter of hundreds of valuable pigs and the disbursement of costly shells. In the U.S. people undertake expensive treatments for infertility and an elaborate apparatus of biotechnology is brought in to replace the natural processes where these fail. In both cases the problem of fertility is big business, and biotechnology has come to take the place of rituals, spells, and prayers.

As we have noted, biotechnology also leads to a wide range of ethical problems connected with the definition of parental ties and thus of kinship itself and the rights and responsibilities that flow from it. It also leads to the question of how far it is appropriate for people to control their own reproductive processes. If it is possible by amniocentesis (the use of a surgical needle to take a biopsy from a developing fetus) to determine if the child will suffer from, for example, Down Syndrome (Rapp 1993), this raises the ethical problem of whether or not to terminate the pregnancy. If parents can choose the sex of their offspring, as biotechnology now in principle allows them to do, should they have that right and how will their choices affect demographic patterns and hence eventually sex ratios and marriage possibilities? Of course, people have attempted ritually to influence the sex of children born in many cultures; patterns of infanticide, usually female infanticide practiced for population control or for other reasons, also severely affect demography. Biotechnology has now simply made possible processes that people have desired and magically simulated or earnestly prayed for in the past, and still do, in all parts of the world.

The debates on the new issues created by biotechnology sometimes miss this point, that the drive to control the pathways of reproduction is very ancient and persistent. Further, it is sometimes claimed that biotechnology leads to entirely new notions about the definition of kinship and therefore to fundamental conundrums in the ordering of familial life. While our examples do show that certain elements of the situation brought about by biotechnology are new, for example the creation of a split within the category of genetrix/biological mother, other elements are not new. The general idea that parenthood may belong to more than one mother and father is in fact fundamental to many kinship systems in which classificatory forms of relationship are recognized. More specifically people may distinguish between social and genealogical or biological parenthood. Students in introductory classes to anthropology learn about the case of the Nuer people of the Sudan, among whom social paternity was created by the payment of cattle in bridewealth, but physical paternity might still be recognized or claimed and marked by separate payments to the mother of a child; or the even more striking point that a woman might "marry" another woman to the name of her dead husband, so that sons might be affiliated to him and continue his lineage, an arrangement that required both a gender switch and an extra genitor to produce the child (Evans Pritchard 1940, 1951).

The Pacific area is full of examples of what have been called transactions in parenthood, loosely glossed by the English language concept of adoption (Brady 1976), by which elements of parenthood are shared out or exchanged among people, not necessarily in terms of the extinction of one party's set of rights in favor of another's. Indeed it is the tendency in the legal systems of western countries to select a model of adoption that transfers rights from the genetic to the adoptive parents, a practice which leads to severe legal quandaries when the definition of what is genetic itself becomes confused. This model of adoption was selected in order that the complete bundle of parental rights and roles should belong only to the adoptive parents and thus the child would not experience a split sense of affiliation. Yet it often does in fact lead to such a sense when a child discovers that it has been adopted; or if the biological parent later wishes to seek the child out. This in turn is because of the initial, or basic, definition of western kinship in biological or genetic terms. When these terms themselves become moot because of biotechnological advances, a confusion of legal and personal categories is created, which is still being worked out in the case-law of disputes.

By comparison the more flexible and wide-ranging ideas that underpin concepts of kinship in many other societies preclude such an acute form of the problem of affiliation from emerging. Kinship statuses can be more widely shared and parcelled out and can also change over time. Ideas of nurture are as much involved as those of blood, and the interplay between nurture and blood leads to the possibility of flexible affiliations (A. Strathern 1973, Meigs 1989). Even more strikingly, we can point out that the idea of cloning, which has raised philosophical questions not only about kinship in western societies but about the very definitions of individual personhood and identity since the creation by a Scottish biologist of the cloned sheep Dolly, is in certain ways anticipated in the thought of tribal peoples such as those of the Pacific and New Guinea.

Here is the meaning of our title for this section of the chapter. As was pointed out long ago by the armchair anthropologists of the nineteenth and early twentieth centuries who classified customs under headings, the principle of "part for whole" (synecdoche) explains the logic of much magical thought and practice. We present here some examples from the Papua New Guinea Highlands.

—In Pangia , pieces of hair, nail clippings, excrement, or saliva on food fragments may be surreptitiously obtained from a person's body and sent to a distant sorcerer who then places them near a fire or over a pool inhabited by a spirit and manipulates them so as to cause the person's illness or death. This is called *nakenea*, "eaten" (see Ch. 6).

—In Hagen, the *min* or spirit/lifeforce of a person is thought to inhabit every part of a person's body. When people wished in the past to lop off a finger in grief for the death of a kinsperson or spouse they would first mark the finger with a mock blow of the axe in order to warn the *min* to depart from it. The *min* runs away into the bush and is annoyed, and later may take revenge by striking the person at their death (Strauss 1962). The severed finger is a synecdochal person.

—Among the Kewa people of the Southern Highlands Province a folktale records how clan warriors were regenerated from their bones and hair when these were placed into the fire-baskets in the long-house previously occupied by their clansmen (LeRoy 1985:213).

—In a Hagen folktale the man Kaukla goes under a lake searching for his deceased wife in the land of the dead. His sister, who died previously, tells him to let a part of the blood from a finger he had cut off in grief drop onto some vegetables. The sister feeds the vegetables to the dead wife, who is restored to life and goes back with her husband to the land of the living (A. Strathern 1977 pp. 79–80, Vicedom 1943–8 vol.3, myth no. 62).

The first example shows how a part of a person may be operated on to kill that person at a distance. The second indicates that a portion of lifeforce may be in a finger and may even be split off from the person and acquire an agency of its own if it is lopped off. The third reveals that a whole person may be regenerated from a part when it is placed in a ritually powerful location. The fourth also instances regeneration: when a husband's blood is given to his dead wife in food, she comes to life again, with the help of the man's sister.

In a further example from the Duna area, we see again the power of blood:

—Among the Duna there is an idea that a witch who wants to kill and eat a person comes at night and extracts amounts of blood which she/he places in containers and hides in a tree. The "phials" of blood grow and become like the person. When the witch sees this has happened she calls others to join in the feast, and kills and eats the victim.

Here the same logic shows as in the Hagen case, that blood contains lifeforce, and in addition a piece of blood can be "cultured" and grown into a whole simulacrum of the person, who is then available for killing and consumption.

The logic that informs these cases is one that is close enough to the idea of cloning for us to say that these New Guinea peoples have in their imagination anticipated what scientists have now begun in practice to do. It is this same kind of logic, in turn, that informs some of the curative, as opposed to destructive magic that they perform, when they take a substance or item and utter a spell over it or perform a ritual designed to give it the power to overcome sickness in a patient. In their pursuit of fertility and health they have certainly shown that they have a fertile imagination and an aptitude for what we have discussed in chapter nine as imaginal performance.

In this chapter we have counterposed notions from contemporary contexts of biotechnology with ideas and practices from personalistic systems of medicine and cosmic worldviews, pointing to some surprising concordances of themes as well as to obvious differences. We continue to pursue this dual perspective in the next chapter, on physician-patient communication.

Chapter 12

Doctors and Patients:
Communication

Pliskin's study of therapeutic encounters between Israeli doctors and Iranian patients in Israel, as discussed in Chapter Eight, points to many of the problems that belong in complex ways to this topic (Pliskin 1987). She highlights the cultural, intercultural, interactional, and professional elements that impinge on these encounters, making it quite clear that the influence of cultural ideas is very strong and can lead to misunderstanding and miscommunication. Her interethnic example foregrounds a possibility that is always present in all doctor-patient encounters, that communication and/or sympathy between the parties may fail, a possibility that compounds the inherent difficulties of achieving accurate diagnosis and treatment. In other words, the major point to remember here is that a visit to the doctor is not a neutral event, and is not solely guided by scientific considerations in the case of biomedicine, or religious ones in the case of ritual healing. Each side brings to the encounter a great array of considerations, some expressed, some not expressed, which strongly influence the encounter itself. Research in this arena attempts to make clear some of the parameters that influence communication and decision making by doctors and patients by means of direct observation, recording and transcribing, or structured interviews with both patients and doctors.

In this chapter, as in others, we follow the tenets of the "new" ethnopsychiatry as advocated by Atwood Gaines (Ch. 8) by placing biomedical practices and ideas *alongside* those from other contexts and traditions, recognizing both that biomedicine as a general category has its own cultural logic and that this logic is inflected locally in many different ways around the world. (See also here Lock and Gordon 1988.) We do so also in order to subvert the idea that biomedicine is uniquely scientific and neutral in its approach to sickness, although we acknowledge the impressive and sincere attempts made within it to reach a purely scientific and neutral stance. And while biomedicine has its own special logic, this does not mean that other systems lack logics of their own, or even that there is a necessary conflict or difference between the logics involved.

In addition, the topic of medical communication is obviously one that is important to everyone, since all of us suffer some illness and are obliged to seek help for it. The topic is therefore an emotive one, since each person brings to it a fund of personal experiences that are often strongly tinged in positive or negative ways. In biomedical contexts, physicians are important to us and are seen differently from lawyers or accountants because they deal with us at the level of our bodies as well as our minds or our finances. The same tends to be true in other medical regimes also; for example we have seen earlier (Ch. 8) how moral and religious issues deeply surround issues of sickness in Haiti (Brodwin 1996). Embodiment theory has taught us that the most complex social and cultural issues are often encoded at the bodily level. Medicine therefore is bound to touch on and reverberate with these issues.

Research in cross-cultural contexts by anthropologists has shown that the kind of superficial contrasts we might be inclined to make between biomedicine and other systems of medicine do not hold. It is not the case, for example, that in biomedical encounters there is a concentration only on the condition and not on the patient, while in spiritual or spiritualist modes of healing it is the other way around. Rather, in all contexts there is a mixture of factors and thus of what we call curing and healing. The physician may be attempting to assess the patient as a whole while asking questions only about the condition and its symptoms. The religious healer may assume that he or she already knows about the patient either because the patient is a kinsperson or because spirits have revealed all that needs to be known, and therefore may also ask mostly about the condition, as happens in Mexican spiritualist healing (Ch. 7). We must beware, therefore, of setting up false and oversimplified dichotomies here, while recognizing that differences of emphasis do occur.

Nevertheless, we do need to understand that there are different *foci of interest* in different medical systems and these affect the way diagnosis and treatment proceed. In Chapter Four we described some of the traditional foci of interest in the curing activities of Mount Hagen ritual experts (*mön wuö*). The expert might conduct divination to determine if a ghost had attacked the patient, and proceed with a sacrifice to the ghost asking it to let the person go. Here the ghost was seen as "holding the head" of the sick person. Or the expert might declare, after listening to some of the symptoms and the activities of the patient, that it was a bush spirit that had brought the sickness, encouraged by the ghosts of relatives who were annoyed about some moral issue in their sphere. In that case the correct treatment was to ask the bush spirit politely to go away. In such a world of ideas it is understandable that the expert would not need to conduct a physical examination or ask for a medical history. He might, however, ask which kin of the patient were dead and if there were any social obligations not met that might have engaged the negative interests of ghosts. This kind of context is implicitly present in Mexican spiritualist healing, but is also taken for granted. The healer goes into a trance and is informed by her own good spirit which bad spirits may be causing sickness in the patient. The healer's world view also rules out attributions of witchcraft which may come strongly into play elsewhere in explanation of deaths from sicknesses that will not yield to treatment.

Further, in all contexts the doctor/healer has an already existing *framework of ideas and knowledge* that constrains his/her approach to communication. This is self-evident from what has been said above.

Finally, both doctor and patient belong to *particular social contexts* that place them in relation to each other in terms of education, social ties, class, aspects of culture, and the like, a point stressed in the critical medical anthropology approach (see Ch. 13).

Given these three factors (foci of interest, framework of knowledge, and social context), each therapeutic encounter is a negotiated process, marked also by contests or demonstrations of power on either side, since the three factors are also resources that produce power or lack of power to determine decisions that are made and how/why these are followed or not followed by the patient (see Waitzkin 1991). There is therefore a universal set of circumstances that informs the practices of communication that arise here, for example, the ratio between implied and explicit forms of communicative practice varies with the degree of familiarity or distance between the doctor and the patient.

In many contexts of practice the problem of failed communication does not arise very overtly. It does arise, however, in biomedicine, since the doctor is dependent on the patient to give some information that is relevant to diagnosis. It may also arise in part because either doctor or patient may underestimate the problems involved in the process of communication. Biomedicine is based on a distinction between symptoms (reported by patients) and true causes of disease (to be determined by tests). Over-reliance on one or the other side of the diagnostic picture may lead to inaccuracies or implausibilities since similar symptoms can result from different causes, and some symptoms are unlikely to even relate to certain causes, as when a physician requests tests for melanoma on the basis of a patient reporting a sore rib or pulled muscle.

Gilbert Lewis points out another dimension of interest here when he remarks on "the significance of an illness for the individual" (Lewis 1993:104). Starting from the viewpoint that behavior in illness is socially constructed and noting the widely used distinction between disease and illness, in which disease refers to the biomedical domain while illness refers to the experiential domain of patients, he goes on to say that "illness can single someone out. From an individual point of view, a diagnostic label provides only partial identification.... Each illness is unique; it comes at a particular time.... It is an episode in someone's life, part of his or her unique personal history" (p. 104). He goes on to illustrate the point with two case histories from his fieldwork in Papua New Guinea with the Gnau people of Sandaun (West Sepik) Province. In one a senior man has a headache and sits in his house brooding over it. He thinks his maternal kin may have been cutting down a tree on their land. The sister's son is like a tree that grows on the mother's land, and if such a tree is cut down the sister's son may feel pain. A mother's brother has power to call on his ancestors and put a spell on the tree and the sister's son becomes ill. This is a classic case of the logic of imagery and the association between morality and illness, for a mother's brother would do this only if he had a grievance. The sufferer had dreamed of his maternal kin and asked them to spit red betelnut-juice over him (as a possible cure). Next day he was better. In the second case the wives of two brothers fought over a sago palm. The younger brother's wife ran off to her natal home, declaring she was ill. The mother of the two brothers developed a chest infection, and blamed this on the quarreling and disharmony between the two wives. Maybe a spirit of her husband's lineage had made her ill.

The two cases obviously show that a diagnosis of headache or chest infection with no further imputation of social causes would be quite incomplete from the viewpoint of the Gnau. They might well accept biomedical treatment but would still argue that without the social diagnosis and a return to harmony the treatment would not work. They might also be quite correct in this regard given the well-known association between a rise in stress between persons and a weakening of the immune system. Underlying the specificities of Gnau culture there is therefore a broader point: that diagnosis may indeed need to take social context into account simply to improve therapy, i.e. to join curing with healing. Hence communication between doctors and patients might well need to include some social reference, even though the logic of biomedicine itself tends to focus on establishing what condition of disease a patient has.

Even from this latter viewpoint the issue of communication remains crucial, especially in situations where diagnosis is difficult as in the case of angina, or more broadly, cardiovascular conditions in which the symptoms of pain associated with the condition, while usually recognizable as such, may be referred to other parts of the body such as the arms and legs. The patient's report of symptoms needs to be attended to closely for clues as to the condition, which may then be established through angiography. The time a physician spends in discussion with the patient may be important in this regard, although a physician with good rapport and a good technique of enquiry can complete a sound diagnosis in a shorter time period than another lacking these capacities. In life-threatening situations such as liver collapse and organ transplantation, assessing the patient's needs and motivation to survive and recover may also be crucial.

Angina is in fact an appropriate condition to focus on in terms of doctors' communicative and diagnostic practices, for a number of reasons. The term angina covers a variety of specific problems and tends to be reported in different ways by patients. It is, however, recognized to be an insidious and potentially hidden condition that can lead to serious ischemic heart disease, which can be costly to treat and life-threatening if undiagnosed. The word angina itself was first used by William Heberden in 1768 (Pantano 1990:9), and it was initially not considered to be a common condition. Pantano, who studied in the School of Medicine at Pittsburgh (1990:50ff.), points to many of the difficulties in diagnosis. He cites a case where the only symptom experienced was a "lump in the throat" interpreted by the patient as an "attack of nerves." In other cases the pain may be referred to the arm, elbow, or wrist or the lower jaw. In an earlier passage he records the communicative problems that arise in diagnosis:

.... "My head goes into a whirl as I try to remember how John refers to his angina. I glance at my notes, hoping for a quick cue.... Seeing nothing, I flash through my catalog of words and phrases that other patients have used to describe what they are feeling when angina strikes... One lady called it her "elephant" and one man even called it his "little friend"... "That stuff," I finally say and John gets my meaning" (Pantano 1990: 10–11). Similar experience is recounted by Legato and Colman in their study of heart disease as it affects women (1991). They write:

"Angina means different things to different people. Some people experience classic angina —a heaviness, burning or squeezing in the chest, often radiating to the back, up to the neck, and sometimes down the left arm. However... the variations can often be very confusing. For example, I recently saw a forty-nine year old woman who had for several years complained of chronic pain in her jaw" (Legato and Colman 1991: 74).

In this instance the diagnosis of angina was made by investigating more closely the type of pain experienced: a sharp twinge rather than the chronic ache of toothache. The writers ask why the condition took so long to diagnose and answer that it is because many other conditions mimic those of angina (ibid.).

The chief problem seems therefore to be that angina can sometimes be incorrectly diagnosed as a relatively harmless condition. Helman (1994: 15) provides one reason why confusion may arise in the communicative process: the patient may equate the heart with the whole thoracic region. In angina, also, the type of stenosis and its location determine the seriousness of the condition, and accurate assessment may depend on angiography. Angina is a painful and disturbing condition and is likely to produce consultation with a doctor. The patient may also, however, have a drive to consider the condition as *not* serious or life-threatening, thereby modifying the account given to the doctor. Overall, then, angina is a serious condition, in relation to which diagnostic problems can arise, and is therefore appropriate as the focus for an investigation into communicative practices (see also Julian et al. 1982).

We noted above that one of the difficulties in the diagnosis of angina has to do with ambiguities in reports by patients regarding the pains they experience. Indeed, the character of pain is intrinsically subjective and therefore the problem of pain in general raises hard issues of interpretation and action in the doctor-patient communication process (Good et al. 1992).

The question of what one does in general to deal with pain and if one needs to treat all pain has been raised in a number of arenas, one of which is premenstrual syndrome (PMS) which is a condition of pain associated with mood swings that many women experience on monthly intervals prior to menstruation. A debate has arisen over the issue of whether the biological phenomenon should be considered a condition that should be pharmaceutically treated or whether it should simply be recognized as a natural part of the the female's reproductive cycle that does not need to be ignored but perhaps does not need to be hormonally treated either. Although some have suggested that PMS should be chemically treated this may be driven more by desire for pharmaceutical companies to fill a perceived area of need in order to increase revenues as it has so effectively done in the area of anti-aging vitamins, creams, and assorted medicines than a desire to treat a serious illness. The realities of the pain that some women experience as part of their normal cyclical pattern of existence cannot be denied and in some instances associated clinical conditions such as endometriosis (an abnormal condition in which sections of uterine tissue are displaced and can produce severe abdominal cramping for women prior to and during menstruation) do produce excessive pain which can be treated. Individual parameters of pain tolerance and perceptions of what is a normal and abnormal amount of discomfort/pain can only be measured by the individual herself. But the expression of pain is often culturally conditioned, especially in instances of repetitive pain such as that experienced during menstruation or in the experience of birthing which many women encounter repeatedly during their lifetime (see Finkler 1991, 1994c).

Pain, as we have remarked, is a difficult topic to discuss because of the highly subjective nature by which it is perceived. Even though pain can be measured in various ways including monitoring heart rate, blood pressure, or measuring neurological alterations such as changes in neurotransmitter levels, it is difficult to measure individual tolerance and/or acceptability of pain. In some instances what might be described as painful to one person could be described as pleasurable to another. Also, emotionally produced sensations of pain such as those during grieving can be as "painful" to the body as any other painful sensation such as cutting the foot. All of these issues may emerge in discussions between doctors and patients, as the various cases explored in Good et al. 1992 demonstrate (e.g. Byron Good's study of Brian, a twenty-eight year old man who suffered chronic pain labeled as TMJ, tempero-mandibular joint syndrome, and Paul Brodwin's study of Diane Reden, a young women with a variety of bodily pains who used her pain symptoms like a language to communicate with others, including her physicians).

How can studies of communicative and decision-making practices help doctors in their work of caring for patients and treating their conditions? In order to answer this question, it is necessary to study the practices of physicians themselves as the objectified results of certain basic tenets that have grown up within biomedicine. Adherence to these tenets remains strong in practice because they are built into the rules by which doctors are expected to go about their business. This is particularly true in the sphere of decision making. The formal logic by which biomedicine operates entails (a) a distinction between symptoms and causes; (b) the causes involved belong to the category of disease-bearing pathogens; (c) causes are hidden from the patient and can be identified only by the doctor; (d) if such causes cannot be found, the matter is out of the doctor's sphere of investigation. Further, a physician's rule of thumb operates in terms of rule-out procedures, by which the doctor first tests for a more serious condition, then if this is ruled out proceeds to less serious possibilities. Here serious is defined as life-threatening. There are two dangers with this kind of procedure, well established as it is: (1) it is likely to upset the patient, sometimes quite unnecessarily; (2) if the test for a serious condition proves negative, the doctor may lose interest or run out of ideas on how to regard the patient's condition. In either case, there are costs in terms of patient noncompliance or patient distress. It is precisely at the boundary between "disease" and "illness" that such counterproductive effects may be found.

Another problem arises from reliance on machines for diagnostic purposes. Machine-based tests are of obvious value in rule-out procedures. However, a particular test can usually exclude only one or a few possibilities, and it may give no positive indications to aid further diagnosis. Machines should *not* be made to function instead of the decision-making responsibility on the part of the doctor. It is of interest therefore to see how the human/machine interface operates in doctors' diagnostic practices.

The questions to be asked in inquiries of this sort would include ones aimed at producing evidence for (a) the doctor's picture of how diagnosis of a particular condition proceeds, (b) the breadth or narrowness of the doctor's conception of the condition, (c) the degree of reliance on machine-based tests, and (d) the degree of persistence in following up conditions. Success in diagnosing and treating certain conditions depends in fact on broadening rather than narrowing the doctor's decison-making processes; and communicative factors are crucial in this process of broadening the doctor's perception of the patient's condition.

An arena in which doctor-patient communication is crucial is that of chronic conditions which require lifelong maintenance procedures. One such condition is diabetes. Approximately eleven million Americans or 5% of the U.S. population are estimated to have diabetes mellitus. African-Americans and Hispanics are at higher risk of developing the disease than other groups, and a common form of diabetes (gestational diabetes) occurs in 3–5% of pregnant women. The management of diabetes is complex, involving the adherence to a prescribed diet, exercise regimen, and/or hypoglycemic medication. The management process is facilitated when patients and physicians are able to exchange information and rely on each other in a relationship of communication and mutual understanding.

The concept of controlling the body through a deliberate discipline may be one that is unfamiliar to patients or difficult for them to execute because of pressures from family situations, neighborhood factors, economic demands, or other interacting forces. Physicians in training must learn to understand the illness narratives provided to them in terms of a patient's cultural and ethnic milieu. These narratives may be highly coded and in need of elaborate unpacking. Illustrations of this can be found in a study of the process of diabetic consultation in an urban American public clinic, Chicago's Cook County Family Practice Clinic [Fantus] (Stewart and Strathern 1997). This clinic accepts both scheduled patients with appointments and walk-in patients who come from diverse neighborhoods in Chicago. The clinic attempts to provide a sense of patient-physician continuity by matching patients whenever possible with the same physician on as many visits as possible. The research study included an exploration of doctor talk (i.e., the discourse between medical students/junior physicians [residents] in training and their senior physician supervisors [attendings]). This medical student/resident interaction with attending physicians is part of a training program at Cook County Hospital and the medical student's/resident's performance during this exchange is evaluated by the attending. During these sessions the attending physician also acts in the capacity of a mentor. Robert Hahn in *Sickness and Healing* reports on his interviews with Barry Siegler, M.D., an established physician who had been interacting with patients for many, many years. Siegler stated that 90% of what a physician knows comes from experience with patients after the training of formal education that occurs in the structured framework of medical school (Hahn 1995: 181). The program at Cook County is hoping to transfer some of the knowledge gained through on the job experience of senior physicians to medical students/residents who are just beginning to learn about these parameters of the profession.

Physicians and patients often hold discrepant models of health and illness that may affect the effectiveness of communication during the clinical visit. These discrepancies can arise when certain aspects of the patient's illness are not well defined within existing biomedical paradigms, such as when various factors that affect control of diabetes mellitus are not well understood and are manifested in unpredictable ways in different individuals. An example of this is the way that hormonal shifts that occur in the female monthly cycle transmogrify management regimens.

In the study, recorded notes were kept of observations on the reports of students/residents with attending physicians. The reports were given to the attendings immediately after the medical student/resident had examined the patient and conducted the patient interview. The patient was asked to wait while this report was being given. After the attending had listened and made whatever comments he thought were appropriate, the medical student/resident revisited the patient in the examination room and at that point wrote prescriptions, gave advice, and completed his/her interaction with the patient.

The medical interview is conducted as a means to obtain information. The whole process is completed to some degree for an audience of other physicians who will not only make decisions based on the documented case, but judge the student/resident based on his/her work. Often there is a conscious editing out of patients' stories in an effort to detail what is thought to be the important information. "What you need to present to me (the attending physician) is the stuff we're going to work on" (Good 1994: 78). But how this is determined is a difficult process of decision making. The patient as case is presented as a genre of story telling through which persons are formulated and reformulated as medical problems. The learning of what "the important stuff" to relate is and how to present this information in a persuasive way is central to becoming a physician.

Some cases will illustrate these processes:

Case A:

A fourth year medical student's report to the attending physician explains that "the diabetic patients that I see do not understand diabetes. They only see a series of complications that arise from having diabetes. Patients have heard of the disease (diabetes) and they do know that it can cause chronic problems. Patients are given a schedule listing amounts of insulin and times that it should be taken. This schedule is not to be modified without the consultation with the physician."

In this instance we see that the patient is presented by the student as being ignorant about his/her condition. Also the patient is presented as passive and highly dependent on the physician for even minor alterations in diabetic regime. This image is one that negates the patients' ability to learn how to adjust their insulin dosages in response to changing factors in their lives and denies any agency to the patient in his/her control of the condition.

Case B

An Asian American medical student's report on a fifty-one year old male patient.

The patient had recently been seen at the emergency room at 4:30 a.m. for a hypoglycemic attack (dangerously low blood sugar levels) and had been subsequently referred to the clinic for adjustment of his insulin regime in order to avoid further attacks of this sort.

After listening to the comments of the medical student the attending physician reminded the student to review the signs of hypoglycemia with the patient. In response to this admonition, the student said that he assumed the patient knew what the signs of hypoglycemia were since he had had diabetes for twenty-two years. The attending pointed out that the physician should ask rather than make assumptions about what the patient knows.

Furthermore, the attending physician recommended that the medical student inquire about the patient's family, asking if the patient's wife could be more involved in making sure that the patient ate his meals at the appropriate times since the patient was sometimes not eating his dinner and not following other aspects of his diet plan.

Case C

An African-American female resident's report on a fifty-four year old female Native American patient.

The patient routinely had high blood sugar levels on testing at her scheduled visits in the clinic. When questioned about this hyperglycemia the patient explained that it was produced by stress and anxiety as a result of her thirteen year old daughter's behavior. Here the patient is describing the lack of control that she has over her social relationships and the effect that these relationships have on her health. She also admitted to following her diet plan loosely and eating high sugar food such as cake without altering her insulin intake thereby blaming her own actions in addition to those of her daughter.

The resident recommended increasing the patient's insulin in general for tighter control. The attending provided no further recommendations. In reporting this patient's history to the attending it was evident that the resident had used the patient's chart to gather information about the patient more than she had put questions to the patient or listened to the patient's narrative of her illness.

In these three instances we can see that different students/residents each had very different styles and ways of interacting with patients. Usually there was not a strong relationship with the patient and a lack of consideration of family support systems was prevalent. The attending in one case, however, drew attention to this dimension.

These three instances suggest in general the following points: (1) attention should be paid to perceived disparitites of knowledge and viewpoint between physician, student, and patient; (2) a picture of the patient's agency and of how to enhance it needs to be formed by physician and student; (3) patients' understandings of the two-way interactive process between diet, insulin intake, and blood sugar levels need to be explored, including the language of report between student and physician compared to the language of the clinical interview between student and patient; (4) the patient's explanatory model (EM) needs to be matched against that of the physician and student; and (5) the kinds of pointers given by physicians to students, exemplifying their experience as against their technical training, need to be closely scrutinized in terms of how and whether they refer to points (1) and (2) above.

Works on narrative accounts of illness are numerous in the literature (Mischler 1986; Gunnarrson et al. 1995; Good 1994; Finkler 1995) and Mischler has conducted detailed studies of doctor-patient dialogues (1986a and 1986b) in order to better understand the barriers in communication between care givers and care receivers. Waitzkin has analyzed communication in terms of power differentials between doctors and patients (Waitzkin 1991).

Some of the communication difficulties that arise between patients and physicians result from "differences in the speech registers used by doctors compared to that of patients" (Bourhis et al. 1989: 339) This may be a product of various socioeconomic factors. "Knowing something about the ethnographic setting, the perception of and characteristics attributed to others, and broader and local social organizational conditions becomes imperative for an understanding of linguistic and non-linguistic aspects of communicative events" (Cicourel 1992: 294). Byron Good refers to semantic networks that exist between individuals and he stresses that it is essential to translate terms used in medical discourses in order to explore meaningfully related domains of social life and experience, as well as semantic domains (Good 1994: 171–174).

Another difficulty that arises in patient-physician communication is that medical students are in general trained to conceptualize the mind and body as separate entities, thereby establishing an artificial dichotomy. In addition to the mode of medical training received, the value systems of individual medical students and physicians vary greatly and influence how information is transmitted and obtained. Attempting to understand the whole patient and treat the whole person who exists within a complex social nexus is one of the more insightful ways of lessening communication problems. Biomedicine needs to draw upon cosmology, ontology, epistemology, understandings of personhood, society, morality, and religion for its most effective expression (Lock and Gordon 1988).

It is important to stress that the whole patient/person here means the mind-body complex, the focus of much anthropological theorizing and discussion today (e.g. A. J. Strathern 1996). The problem may be that patients themselves do not see themselves in this way: they may see themselves as in some fashion separate from their bodies. Patients may need to integrate the experience of their bodies into their "mindful" pictures of themselves, while physicians may need to integrate a picture of the patient's mind into their view of the patient's body.

The underlying notions of agency entertained by physicians and patients in the intersubjective realm of patient care need to be examined in order to understand better how health care professionals can establish more meaningful exchanges between themselves and their patients to help patients with diabetes. Disease occurs not only in the body, in the sense of an ontological order, but in time, in place, in history, and in the context of lived experience and the social world. Meaning and knowledge are therefore always negotiated in reference to a world constituted in human experience, formulated and apprehended through symbolic forms and distinctive interpretive practices. Thus, integrating the concerns of patients and their life circumstances into holistic treatment regimes seems to be imperative in providing health care.

From the viewpoint of physicians, issues of and research into communicative practices tend to be formulated in terms of "patient compliance or non-compliance" (Singer 1987: 251). Singer takes his stand on the issue of who *should* have power, the physician or the patient, thus identifying his position as within critical medical anthropology (CMA). Clearly such a matter is highly complex and cannot be settled generally. However, we can say that there is always a process of negotiation between the physician and the patient and this is what the communication between them is about. We can also suggest that both sides in the encounter can best make their decisions if the information flow between them is optimal. Singer gives a case history of a woman anxious to have a child before age thirty-five and concerned about her apparent pregnancy (which turned out to be ectopic). The case history is replete with episodes in which the patient, partly because of her high state of anxiety, was left with unanswered questions. On one occasion she was told by her obstetrician "I'm sorry, we have only seven minutes per patient" (p. 257). Singer notes at the beginning of his paper that the condition of ectopic pregnancy is commonly missed by physicians and that the mortality rate if it is undiagnosed is over 60% (p. 249). The subject of the study eventually did deliver a normal baby, but commented that the word patient must be related to patience, "because that's what patients are expected to have" (p. 257). This case study concerned health care undertaken through an HMO, and points out to patients the dangers of a time-centered focus, based on a need for through-put and profit (for general comparative studies on this issue see Franken-berg 1992).

Research can also be focused on physicians themselves. Thomas Maretzki emphasizes out the need to include the physician in "healer-centered research" (Maretzki 1985: 23). In the same volume Robert Hahn gives a complex "portrait of an internist" (Hahn 1985: 51–114) who combines bio-medicine practice with religious attitudes in which Nature takes the place of God, and who reveals all too clearly his emotional feelings, ethical judg-ments, and his own frustration that medicine is an imperfect science. This internist also refuses to rely simply on numerical tests and insists on know-ing a patient's history. Clearly he tends toward the healing rather than the curing end of the spectrum, yet he insists also on concentrating on physi-ological matters and avoiding too much discussion of the patient's "other troubles" (p. 91). The portrait as a whole reveals the dilemmas of bio-medical practitioners at a deep everyday level. The more experienced and engaged they are, the more they know that Gilbert Lewis's aphorism ("each illness is unique") is true. But the professional cultural logic of western biomedicine (WBM) leads them back to physiology and away from so-ciality; whereas cultural diagnosis among the Gnau leads away from phys-iology and to sociality, specifically into the morality of kinship relations.

Pearl Katz, in the same volume as Hahn (Katz 1985: 155ff), quotes the anecdote of a surgeon who is reported to have said "A surgeon knows nothing, but does everything. An internist knows everything, but does nothing." This could be an ironic intertextual comment on the dilemmas of Hahn's internist, Barry. It also points out the *differences* between pro-fessional practitioners within WBM itself. Surgeons see themselves as doing battle and engaging in something like heroics. They tend also to be au-thoritarian and less concerned with communicating matters to the patient. This could lead to confusion Katz comments here: "The decision-making options were made explicit by the surgeon who was willing to make a dif-ficult decision. The decision-making options were made confused by the sur-geon unwilling to make the difficult decision" (p. 169).

This example highlights the overall point of this chapter, that commu-nication is *always* important, and indeed plays an important part in deci-sion making itself.

It can also be important to find something to communicate when ex-tensive batteries of tests fail to reveal a biomedical condition in spite of reported symptoms of illness, as when one of us (AJS) was told by a young doctor, after looking over a thick dossier of test results: "We can't find anything. Now go away and be well." The advice was heeded.

The publications from the 1980s have been followed by over a decade of continuing work focusing on patients, physicians, and communication patterns of primary care physicians (e.g. Rotes, Deborah et al. 1997, Laine and Davidoff 1996, and Novack, Dennis H. et al. 1997, all published in the *Journal of the American Medical Association*). Laine and Davidoff, taking off from the CMA approach, explore the implications of the growth of the concept of patient-centered medicine, care that is closely congruent with and responsive to patients' wants, needs, and preferences, and is correspondingly distanced from the older paternalistic model. Yet advice can be given in a "fraternal" or "sororal" way also, as perhaps evidenced by the preceding personal anecdote, and can be valuable in its own right. Within the medical profession there are reassessments of modes of reasoning in clinical practice (Higgs and Jones 1995, Tanner 1993); and an issue of the *Medical Anthropology Quarterly* (1998, 12(3)) contains five papers exploring anthropological dimensions of physicians' reasoning compared with that of patients (including narrative and moral dimensions as well as the issue of decision-making models and different versions of rationality).

Chapter 13

Critical Medical Anthropology

Critical medical anthropology (CMA) has emerged as a means to set a theoretical framework around the contributions from anthropological studies of healing and curing practices. This framework attempts to fit medical anthropological findings into the political and economic situations of their particular cultural arenas. The approach contextualizes ethnographic data in terms of the mix of political and economic pressures that are involved in shaping social behavior and generating social meanings. The aim of critical medical anthropology is to understand better how medical/healing practices are regulated and, in some instances, to help evaluate the terms in which health services are provided with an eye to improving availability and effectiveness of health care. The approach developed from concern over the impact of capitalism on global health care, the inequalities in the availability of medical resources, and the influence of Western biomedical practices over local ones.

Some have criticized CMA for focusing too heavily on global social relationships and their dependency upon capitalism. Irwin Press suggests that these models direct the explanations for problems in medical systems to large-scale social and economic factors only (Press 1990). He concedes that this may illuminate to some extent the availability and overall organization of some arenas of medical care, but he points out that the method provides little insight into the microlevel organization of the system, such as the communication difficulties that arise between patients and physicians (see Ch. 12). Others such as Merrill Singer have suggested ways in which critical medical anthropology's findings might be used in order to effect changes in practices of health care systems through the implementation of specific programs.

The problems, as well as the appeal, of the CMA approach reside in a general programmatic problem in contemporary anthropological work. At times in the past, anthropologists tended to describe small-scale, isolated cultures as independent units without systematically setting these into a broader historical context. This is in itself only partially true, but in any case the practice has long disappeared and broad contexts are very much in evidence in anthropologists' accounts, although many anthropologists would agree that our main strength still lies in explicating local contexts. The problem nowadays is specifically how to combine interpretive work with political economy analyses (Marcus and Fischer 1986; Knauft 1996). CMA aims to approach the problem from the macrolevel of political economy, looking at how the larger picture affects the smaller, and then how meanings may be generated in the process of historical influence. As Gaines has argued (see Ch. 8 in this book), the approach tends to downplay the agency of people themselves and their ability to create their own meanings from, and solutions to, the problems of sickness.

In a recent textbook on the CMA approach, Baer, Singer, and Susser devote a central part of their exposition to the health problems associated with homelessness, addictions to alcohol and smoking, the use of illicit drugs, and AIDS, the last of which they call "a disease of the global system" (Baer, Singer and Susser 1997: 159). In all of these contexts their concern is to show that the exercise of political and economic power in decision making wields a significant influence on health patterns of the masses. Hence social scientists cannot avoid making statements that in one way or another are connected to these spheres of politics and economics, and there is also no such thing as a neutral or value-free social science. Atwood Gaines would doubtless agree with the general proposition, adding that in the interpretive approach more stress is placed on people's active choices and less on the large coercive frameworks that constrain these choices. In principle it is obvious that both approaches have their strengths and limitations (see also McElroy 1996 for a defense of medical ecology approaches).

CMA tends to focus on the material results of people's actions, whether freely chosen or coerced. With regard to tobacco smoking in the industrialized countries, for example, Baer, Singer, and Susser correctly point out that it is linked to coronary heart disease, lung cancer, and chronic obstructive pulmonary disease (1997: 103),and they add a long list of other conditions including various cancers. The World Health Organization in 1994 estimated that around the world three million people die each year from diseases brought on through the use of tobacco. Knowledge about tobacco's deleterious effects is not new, yet the tobacco industry, by paying for advertisements, keeps its sales up, and young people are inducted into the smoking habit (although in the United States there has been a presidentially-sponsored campaign against the targeting of teenagers in advertisements during 1997 and 1998). The process of criticism and defense of smoking has been going on since 1602, when the first known tract against smoking was published in England (Baer, Singer, and Susser 1997: 107). Governments, however, found it useful to tap into the income produced from tobacco sales by levying taxes on them, and so tobacco was transformed into a source of revenue accumulation and thus a force in history. Concomitantly, the methods of its production were streamlined and automated over time, enabling greater output and thus greater consumption.

The state tobacco monopoly in China produces in excess of 1.5 trillion cigarettes per year, which are all smoked in China itself. By the year 2000 it is predicted that in China alone more than two million people will die of tobacco-related diseases per year. Baer, Singer, and Susser also argue that the tobacco industry in America targets Hispanics and African Americans (p. 111), and cite the explanation that smoking serves as an anticipatory rite of passage into mainstream or adult status for members of subordinated social categories such as minorities (they include youth and women here). This explanation can in fact be generalized beyond the category of minorities, by pointing out that smoking will be adopted whenever and wherever it is an approved form of social recreation within a group, the more so since it is an addictive habit that produces short-term pleasures at the cost of long-term bodily deterioration whenever its incidence rises above some certified level of moderation.

Baer, Singer, and Susser rightly point to the persuasive effects of smoking advertising in Hispanic communities showing young, affluent, light-skinned, and happy people smoking (p. 114). But again, we may say that all advertising depends on this kind of magical contiguity, and it is not only minorities who are prone to magical forms of thinking that can be seen as the basis for associative forms of rituals in New York or London as well as New Guinea (A. Strathern 1993: 30–31). The point is well made in Philip Larkin's poem ironically entitled "Essential Beauty":

> In frames as large as rooms that face all ways
> And block the ends of streets with giant loaves,
> Screen graves with custard, cover slums with praise
> Of motor-oil and cuts of salmon, shine
> Perpetually these sharply-pictured groves
> Of how life should be. High above the gutter
> A silver knife sinks into golden butter...
> (Larkin 1998:144)

Larkin's wry juxtaposition of graves and custards, slums with salmon, and gutters with butter makes the point that advertisements cover up harsh realities, creating an ideal facade of desire on a world of deprivation. The venue might be Hull or Coventry in England, the locale an ordinary working class area. But Larkin does not suggest that anyone is particularly deceived by billboards. However, the supposition that Baer, Singer, and Susser make is that certain minorities are *more vulnerable* than others to advertising campaigns that cynically exploit their aspirations and desires. Perhaps this is correct. Yet minorities also produce strong forms of resistance to the status quo, showing that they are not so easily offered a simulacrum in place of a reality.

The authors use this transition to motivation as a bridge to what we can easily recognize as an interpretive approach by taking a look at anthropological discussions of smoking behavior from the cross-cultural record. At the outset of their chapter on smoking, in fact, they mention the use of tobacco products by Native Americans, recognizing that tobacco cultivation probably originated in South America and that it was "deeply rooted" in the indigenous cultures of many people in New World (p. 103). They argue that its consumption was subject to ceremonial controls and inhalation was not emphasized, hence it may not have been a significant health problem prior to European contact. This is a backdrop to their exposition of the subsequent deleterious effects of capitalism.

However, this contrast between precapitalist and capitalist smoking patterns may not be entirely valid. Anthropologists have widely noted the use of tobacco smoking in sacred rituals. Roy Rappaport, for example, depicts Maring shamanic experts in Papua New Guinea as energetically smoking tobacco, inhaling deeply and rapidly in order to induce in themselves the ability to communicate with a Female Spirit, the Smoke-Woman (*kun kaze ambra*) (Rappaport 1968: 40–41, 119). In Pangia in the Southern Highlands Province of PNG ritual experts who acted as seers able to discern the actions of malevolent water spirits (*uelali*) in causing sickness began their sessions with patients by the vigorous inhalation of tobacco from wooden holders. Thus fortified, they began their inspections. In Amazonia, Wilpert reports an account by Francis Huxley of an Urubu shaman who smoked a cigar by "taking the smoke with great sucking gasps right into his lungs, working his shoulders like bellows to get as much smoke in as possible" (Wilpert 1987: 108 quoting Huxley 1957: 195). These examples suggest that it was precisely the context of ceremonial use that called for the heavy inhalation of smoke, making the practice a health risk for the shamans at least. Smoking as a health risk cannot therefore be attributed only to the capitalist world and its industrial logic; although the replication of such risks can certainly be attributed in this way.

Baer, Singer, and Susser also note that indigenous populations, once introduced to smoking, have often become highly addicted to it, as happened among the Trukese in Micronesia in the 1870s (Marshall 1979: 36). Elsewhere, as in the New Guinea Highlands, it is not clear exactly how tobacco was introduced, but it predated the direct arrival of Europeans in the 1930s, and it may have passed from group to group in the manner that Alfred Kroeber suggested for Native Americans, in cultural packages associated with rituals (Kroeber 1939). Here, then, we find precapitalist ritual entrepreneurs standing in the place of industrial capitalist entrepreneurs. One of the reasons people also give for their adoption of tobacco-smoking is that it brings *benefits* of wellbeing, such as relaxation, sociability, hunger and pain reduction, and better digestion. In other words, in such cases people see tobacco not as a cause of disease but as an antidote for various minor discomforts of life, as a kind of medicine (Baer, Singer, and Susser 1997: 120, with reference to subsistence farmers in South India). One can easily imagine similar reasons being given by New Guinea farmers (of either sex, since women in many Melanesian societies smoked as well as men). In a traditional ballad (*kang rom*) from the Mount Hagen area, a young woman magically spits at a certain point in the story and from her spittle tobacco plants grow: a scene that reflects both the magical powers of the mouth and its substances in association with the female gender, and the possible encoding of a historical fact that tobacco use passed along the pathways of marriage alliances from group to group, notionally carried by the women who moved as wives to their husbands' places bringing with them the powers of creative nurturance and growth in their bodies. In Hagen, the talk that is made to negotiate and arrange a marriage is called in fact *ol ik*, saliva/spittle talk. Tobacco is also traditionally appreciated as a luxury, though its use has recently been banned by charismatic/fundamentalist Christian churches.

Baer, Singer, and Susser conclude their cross-cultural survey of tobacco use by arguing that through tobacco consumption local populations are "locked into the global economic system"(p. 121). While this is true wherever manufactured cigarettes are sold, it is not true of the well-established precapitalist diffusion of tobacco plants in Amazonia and New Guinea. That is, there was a precapitalist phase of diffusion, whose success was also based on tobacco's addictive powers (like those of sugar, tea, and coffee). The CMA approach seems to have led these authors to gloss over this point, which is evident from their account. Further, ritual inhalation of tobacco smoke seems to have been quite important in some precapitalist cases. Ritual regulation, therefore, need not necessarily protect against health hazards; nor, we may add, does social or recreational use of tobacco necessarily lead to severe health hazards, if it is controlled and moderate. Nothing too much, as in the Greek maxim, appears to be the moral here, so that teaching the dangers and the need for restraint in tobacco use might appear to be a logical step to take.

In their own conclusions, however, Baer, Singer, and Susser take a slightly different approach, stressing the need to include in ethnographic studies not only individual, or even collective, behavioral patterns, but also the actions of governments and corporations and the ways in which they argue their cases through the production of meanings and symbols. In a resolution of the supposed antinomy between CMA and interpretive approaches they rightly say that the (proper) purpose of CMA is a "type of integrated study of political economy and cultural meaning"(p. 123). In commenting on their particular study of tobacco use we have simply wished to point to the necessity for as much rigor of thinking on the interpretive as on the

CMA side of the analysis, and to warn against the tendency to use analysis simply as a platform for indicating the evils of capitalism, which can lead to romanticizing the accounts given of the precapitalist world. In spite of this, the CMA approach is one that brings medical anthropology firmly into the sphere of contemporary global relevance and debate on ethical and political issues as well as grounding itself in one branch of mainstream social theory, the critique of capitalism. This mode of analysis can both illuminate social trends and provide pointers for policies. There is a need, however, to look carefully at all sides of any issue. While social science can never be value-free, it does not have to be directly adversarial. Rather, its major contribution is to enlighten discussion with balanced reviews of issues. It is notable here that, at the end of their review of the problem of AIDS, Baer, Singer, and Susser also introduce a humanistic element, saying that "it is vital we remain sensitive to the individual level of experience and action" and that the goal of the CMA is to help create "a more humane health care system and more humane lives for all people"(p. 188). Few would disagree in principle with such broad ideals, which go well beyond the specific theoretical gambits customarily employed in either political economy or interpretive analyses as such, reaching rather to the level of *humani nihil a me alienum puto*.

Chapter 14

Conclusions: Curing and Healing

The main aims of this book have been (1) to give a conspectus of the arenas of thinking in medical anthropology, seen largely from the cultural viewpoint, and (2) to weave into this conspectus the general distinction which has become foundational to the cultural approach in medical anthropology, the distinction between disease and illness. Putting these themes into global perspective has also meant that we have chosen ethnographic examples from around the world, although many of our cases have been drawn from Asia and the Pacific, areas with which we are familiar. As explained in the Introduction, we have also concentrated on giving our examples and case-histories in some detail rather than attempting brief mentions of materials from a very large number of contexts. We have done this in order to follow the anthropological maxim that contextualizing data is important. Overall, the goal has been to make the book usable for general discussions in medical anthropology, while also working into it some of our own analytical concerns that we think are especially significant at the research level (for example our survey of the importance and scope of humoral ideas of the body outside of Latin America as well as within it, and the importance of Thomas Csordas's cultural phenomenology approach to the topic of ritual healing).

The mention of Csordas's work brings us to our chief purpose here, which is to review the discussions on the distinction between curing and healing that appear throughout the book. This distinction can be seen as (1) a classificatory tool, (2) an interpretive tool, and (3) a tool for assisting in the comparison and explanation of therapeutic systems. It can also be brought to bear on issues having to do with medical pluralism.

Curing vs. Healing as a Classificatory Tool

The distinction falls into line with that between disease and illness, so that we can say disease : illness : : curing : healing. Any such formulation

191

runs the risk of oversimplification, but we can use it as a starting point for classifications. Since we have identified biomedicine as concerned largely with disease and with curing, it is reasonable to expect that much of the data on medical systems we have called personalistic might relate to the problems of illness and healing. In looking, therefore, at the introduction of biomedicine into personalistic systems and the pluralistic situation it induces, we might see a shift in perceptions from personalistic/moralistic issues to attributes linked to the curing of diseases.

It would be a mistake, however, to accept such a classificatory scheme wholesale. First, biomedical physicians are becoming increasingly aware of the need to attend to the whole person *in addition to* the specific conditions the person may have, if only because in many cases this approach is the best one to use to effect curing, or at least management of the condition. And biomedical physicians may be aware that the relationship they build up with their patients contributes to therapeutic outcomes. (See Finkler 1994b for a general comparison between biomedicine and sacred healing and Brody 1992 on physician-patient relationships and "the healer's power.")

Conversely, it is also important to realize that ethnomedical systems always involve a mix of curing and healing emphases, so that curing can be found in personalistic/moralistic systems as well as in ones geared to naturalistic and/or biomedical principles. Shamans, medicine men, and ritual experts may all be just as concerned to cure the specific condition (disease) as to heal the whole person. The point, in turn, makes it easy to understand why a symbiotic relationship may develop between biomedicine and other medical traditions, wherever there is mutual respect between them. The goals of medical practitioners may overlap, and one may be happy to refer patients to the other. Most commonly we find that non-biomedical practitioners, recognizing their own limitations, are happy to refer patients to biomedical specialists. In Japan, as we have seen, there is a balanced arrangement of mutual referrals. This is because *kanpo* medicine there carries high status and marks national identity, and its practitioners are also biomedically trained. Such a felicitous situation is less often found elsewhere. In New Guinea, for example, it is more likely that an enthusiastic adoption of biomedicine is accompanied by an uneasy feeling that it cannot deal with local syndromes such as sorcery or pollution, and covert pluralism emerges.

In the therapeutic system of North American Charismatic Catholics we found a linking of curing and healing in a manner reminiscent of Papua New Guinea. What they call physical healing (our curing) may depend on a prior inner healing (our healing). This is equivalent to our saying that patients' attitudes are crucial in the therapeutic process. It is also equivalent to saying that patients must "cast out anger" or "achieve a balanced state of mind" (compare Kleinman 1988: 108–141, addressing the question "how do psychiatrists heal?").

From this we see that perhaps more interesting than the simple classificatory model of distinction is the idea that we should focus on the *interplay* between elements of curing and healing found in a given medical system.

Curing and Healing:
An Interpretive Tool

As implied above, we can use the distinction to pry apart elements of therapeutic encounters and to explore their synergistic or contradictory effects within the overall medical process. We can observe, for example, when and how practitioners switch from one modality to the other, or how they try to combine them. We suggest that a curing approach may be succeeded by a healing one if a condition proves stubborn or difficult to deal with. As the process goes on, the moral forces of the community are likely to be brought more and more to bear on the problem. A good illustration of this is found in the Duna ritual of "striking the pig's nose," at which the female expert would invite the community of kin to hold onto the tethering rope of the pig to be sacrificed.

In looking at humoral ideas in the Latin American context we have also seen that naturalistic ideas may be combined with personalistic ones, and that when this is done moral and spiritual elements are brought into play. Mexican Spiritualist healers deliberately combine moral homilies with medical prescriptions in order to improve their authority over their patients. Where simple prescriptions fail, they may attempt to induct the patient into the communal, moral life of the Temple, in which case the overall context works to heal the sufferer.

In Mount Hagen the curing activities of the *mön wuö* (ritual specialists) have been almost entirely taken over by the biomedical system; whereas aspects of their healing work have been taken over by Christian prayers, especially in the Charismatic churches. This pattern holds also for the Duna people, with the problem that there is thought to be no really effective way of countering witchcraft (Ch. 5). Rather than fears of witchcraft fading away, they actually feed on epidemics and the patterns of death they produce.

Curing and Healing:
A Tool for Comparison and Explanation

If our distinction begins as a classificatory tool and is refined into a means of better understanding the nuances of therapeutic activities, does this help as much when we look again in a broader way at data and try to make some further comparisons between systems? The answer, we think, is yes it can, as one approach among several. First, as noted above, we can look for emphases within a system. Then we can try to correlate these with other cultural and social factors. The biomedical view of curing, for instance, has been convincingly linked to broad historical and cultural aspects of thought and practice in the Western traditions to which it belongs (Lock and Gordon 1988), although case studies show that in practice these broad aspects may be greatly modified in everyday life (Lindenbaum and Lock 1993). Searching for the expression of an emphasis in everyday practice becomes, then, a way of looking at case materials with a view to explaining them.

The same approach can be used to answer questions of why people respond as they do to biomedicine when it is newly introduced into a social context. We return here to our New Guinea examples. A simplistic prediction of the response to biomedicine by these peoples might have been that they would resist it because of their own religious concepts about the world, or that they would adopt it wholesale, throwing aside their previous practices. The reality is much more complex than either of these two predictions, as we have seen. Among the Huli people aid posts are frequented and biomedical treatments are popular, but certain conditions, thought to be caused by witchcraft, pollution, or ghost attack, cannot be handled by biomedicine. Christian prayers may offer some protection, but they also may leave a lacuna. The overall result is a patchwork of conflicting tendencies, an uneven development or profile of changes, that explains the emotions of disturbance and insecurity people feel in parallel with their new acceptance of biomedicine. The situation among the Duna is the same.

In Hagen, among the Melpa speakers, biomedicine is also widely accepted, and currently the concern lies with how to afford it, since pharmacy medicines are costly and visits to the doctor more so, while subsidised hospital medicines are in short supply. Concomitantly, the Hageners are beset with fears of the increase of cannibalistic witchcraft and are turning more and more to the solutions of Charismatic Christianity to produce healing in their lives as a whole. This case shows that the need for curing has to be adequately met. If aid posts do not achieve this, as in 1998 they were failing to do, people turn in their anxieties to worries about income or how to afford treatment. In some instances in the more remote settlements we saw also a return to the use of traditional plant adjuncts, particularly the use of a kind of nettle to irritate the skin and relieve internal pains. People also turn to the churches to meet their needs for security and feelings of identity which their ritual systems as a whole gave them in the past They are looking for a new harmonious balance between curing and healing in their lives.

It is fair to say that our focus in this book has been directed primarily towards healing rather than curing, though by no means exclusively. A reason for this has been the connection between healing and wholeness, senses of personhood and identity that are placed in crisis in situations of abrupt change. Healing itself becomes in this way a tool of cross-cultural analysis, since the search for identity proceeds differently in different cases (see also discussions on embodiment and identity in Good 1994). One study on women as healers in cross-cultural perspective, pursues this viewpoint constructively in terms of gender relations (McClain 1989). Another collection of papers pursues the theme through studies of forms of alternative medicine in America (herbal cures, water cures, homeopathy, osteopathy, chiropractice, Christian Science, and divine healing), all of which involve varying constructions of identity and personhood (Gevitz 1988). We shall illustrate this point further with the example of firewalking, a practice that belongs to Greece but has been adopted also by a movement in America.

Firewalking is regarded in Greece as a very ancient practice whose patron is Saint Constantine. The anthropologist Loring Danforth's book on this topic deals with it as performed by a group of refugees from Thrace, the Kostilides, who settled in the northern part of Greece, Macedonia, in the early 1920s (Danforth 1989:4). The Anastenaria festival among these people involves firewalking and spirit possession, and reaches its climax each year on May 21, the festival of Saints Constantine and Helen. The celebrants consider that Saint Constantine both causes and cures a wide variety of sicknesses; and that he possesses them when they dance and protects them from being burned when they firewalk. Votive offerings, vows, and sacrifices are made to the saint (Danforth 1989: 5). Most of the celebrants are women. Their possession dance enacts a transition from suffering to joy, and gives them roles that empower them, at least ritually, vis-à-vis men. Overall, the festival is said to mark the feelings of community and ancient tradition that give stability and a sense of identity to the Kostilides as a whole in addition to the firewalkers themselves. Danforth, however, takes a further step and compares the Anastenaria among the Kostilides with the firewalking movement, historically derived from the Greek practices, in America. Here the rite of passage, walking across hot coals, remains the same, but the healing experience is expressed somewhat differently. First, it is seen as a ritual of dying and rebirth, and the experience, in the words of one man, is seen as life-changing (Danforth, p. 261): a part of "self-awareness, spiritual transformation, and personal growth" (ibid.). The suffering to joy syndrome is mirrored as a transition from anguish to bliss and a sense of infinity. Furthermore, exponents run workshops and seminars which people pay to attend, with titles such as "Fear into Power: the Firewalk Experience.... Three Steps to Personal Power" (p.

263). It is not very hard to see here echoes of themes that have emerged in our account of religious healing among the Charismatic Catholics of New England in Chapter Nine. The echoes are echoes of what Csordas calls "North American ethnopsychology" in general, and we can clearly see an ideology of self process in different places. In the Macedonian context, the miraculous healings are cures; in the North American cases the healings are framed as healings of the self, indicating growth into an enhanced state and therefore wholeness. But in the Macedonian case this wholeness is expressed collectively, not personally, since each miraculous curing contributes to a collective healing, one that may be particularly important for a group of immigrants transplanted to a new place and in need of claiming a connection with the ancient past as a source of vitality and identity. Physical and personal curing in the Greek case thus translates into collective healing; whereas in the American case the physical firewalking experience, carried out in a collective ritual context, is seen as a means of personal and spiritual healing. This is an example of the productive ways in which curing and healing can be seen as operating differently in different contexts. The concepts thus help to give us leverage on the weighty task of discussing and explaining cross-cultural differences generally.

Questions

Chapter 1

1. What is pluralism and why is it important in studying medical anthropology?
2. How does medical ecology relate to medical anthropology?
3. The authors state that they will present medical anthropology via in-depth ethnographies. In your opinion, will this be more or less useful than the alternative of brief, general, cultural accounts? Why or why not?
4. Illustrate the difference between illness and disease, and healing and curing. What limitations do you foresee with these definitions?
5. How do the authors present the concept of holism? Is this concept an integral part of your accepted "medical system"?

Chapter 2

1. What do the authors mean when they say "actions are bound up with the state of people's emotions, and these in turn are held to influence the state of their bodies"? How does this affect cultural investigations of health and illness?
2. Explain humoral theory. Do you recognize it as logical and pragmatic? Why or why not?
3. How is humoral theory understood with regard to Latin American medicine?
4. What examples do you find illustrate an amalgamation of "culturally mediated ideological beliefs" with regard to concepts of health and illness?
5. Why would it be a good strategy for colonizers to wipe out indigenous forms of medicine?

6. What is the condition of *susto*? What are the symptoms and when does it occur?
7. What are the distinctions between *Kanpo* and biomedicine? Which would you recognize as most efficacious?
8. Why did *Kanpo* or traditional Chinese medicine make a comeback in Japan?
9. What is the concept of *amaeru* and why is it important in the context of Japanese medicine?
10. What is yin and yang? What is *ki*? How do they fit into the framework of Japanese medicine?
11. What is the *Kanpo* definition of health and how is this illustrated in the treatment?
12. How is physiomorphism utilized in Japanese medicine?
13. What similarities/differences do you see between *Kanpo* and Ayurvedic medicine?

Chapter 3

1. How do the Melpa constitue their Humoral System? Describe its processes/functions and how it relates to gender and kinship.
2. What is *noman* and what is its significance with regard to sickness and healing?
3. How does the Melpa Humoral System link emotion and sickness?
4. How is wealth linked with this system, and how is this illustrated in Ongka's presentation of his sickness?
5. How do Yara and Ongka's narratives differ? How would you explain these differences?
6. How does Yara's account link healing with Hagen ideas of identity?

Chapter 4

1. What similarities do you see between the nine spells that are presented? How do the content and images help the spells to work?
2. What "logics" structure the framework for removing spirits?
3. Why is the efficacy of biomedicine so limited with regard to disorders caused by spirit attacks?
4. How and why is social stress linked to belief in the supernatural (witchcraft, second coming of Christ)?

5. How has Christianity changed the regulation and conception of health?

Chapter 5

1. What are the gender dynamics within the practice of witchcraft? In these stories, who are the witches and who is being bewitched?
2. How is witchcraft linked with illness and healing?
3. How does environment factor into illness and healing within the context of witchcraft? Can you draw any conclusions about the people's relationship with the environment?
4. How do blood and consumption of pork factor into these stories?
5. Does sorcery differ from witchcraft? If so, what differences do you see?
6. What is the *tini* among the Duna, and what is its significance in this context?
7. To what extent is the belief in witchcraft pragmatic in explaining the unexplained?

Chapter 6

1. What are the Huli and the Hagen concepts of health and illness? How do morality and social relations factor into each?
2. In what ways does the Huli concept of illness parallel humoral notions of healing?
3. How has Christianity changed concepts of sickness with the Huli? Can Christianity be considered a medical system? Why or why not?
4. How and why has Western medicine been accepted in these cultures? How has it immersed itself in traditional medicine?
5. Outline the three types of Wiru sorcery. Which ones illustrate the most severity in relation to health care?
6. How do you think colonialism affects the physical and mental health situations of the indigenous cultures presented in this chapter? How do medical structures (both indigenous and introduced) relate to the wider forms of culture?

Chapter 7

1. Describe the healing practices that occur in the Spiritualist temples of Mexico. How does health correspond with social interaction?
2. What is the relationship between Spiritual temples and biomedicine? When do you see an amalgamation of both?
3. What characteristics do the Spiritualist healers retain? Why is this important in the ceremony, treatment, and doctor— patient relationship?
4. What explanation can you give for the absence of a patient's verbal statements about his/her condition in the Spiritualist temples?
5. Why would Finkler consider spiritualist treatment a "powerful placebo"? Is this designation correct?
6. Do spiritualist "healings" result in physical and psychological wellness? Do patients accept these treatments as efficacious? How does somatization factor into this process?

Chapter 8

1. Why would culture change make it more difficult for Aboriginal healers to heal?
2. In Pliskin's study, how does the concept of morality play into the physician—patient relationship?
3. What power does sickness give the Aborigines?
4. What are the roles of sorcerers and healers? How can you distinguish between the two?
5. What is *Galka* and how is this ideology important in a communal sense?
6. What does ethnopsychiatry need to take in to account?
7. The authors recognize that "ethnomedical systems are open-ended products of cultural history and are consequently in processes of change." Can this also be said of biomedicine? Why or why not?
8. The authors clarify specific culture-bound syndromes. According to their definition, what could you consider a culture bound syndrome in the U.S.?

Chapter 9

1. What does it mean to be healed within the context of Pentecostal Catholicism?
2. Describe the charismatic healing service.
3. What kind of healing do charismatics stress? How does this parallel the Hagen idea of *Popokl*?
4. What is a protoritual and what are some examples in addition to the ones provided by the authors?
5. What is the role of self processes and imaginal performances in healing? In what other healing/curing circles do these appear? How are they manifested?
6. How are the above processes important for healers?
7. Csordas argues that "self processes are orientational processes in which aspects of the world are thematized," so that the self can further be "objectified as a person with a cultural identity." What does this mean?
8. What is the difference between incremental vs. miraculous healing? Why is this distinction important?

Chapter 10

1. How does the environment play into the humoral scheme of thinking?
2. How do location and economy directly affect health? What are some examples?
3. Why would strangers be more susceptible to fatal disease as opposed to the indigenous community?
4. How does disease change economy?
5. How does colonization relate to disease?
6. Why is it important to look at people's own forms of health-seeking behavior, before attempting to control disease?
7. What are some examples of ethnotheories of disease?
8. In your social context, what diseases are directly related to morality? Why?
9. What is the significance of the story of Haya children growing plastic teeth?

Chapter 11

1. What is the relationship found in some cultural contexts between fertility and the spirit world? Provide some examples. Does this parallel notions of fertility within your own cultural context?
2. How do the causes of infertility relate to social transgression?
3. Give some examples of how women are treated for infertility. What does the treatment tell you about the cultural notions of infertility?
4. What are the gender dynamics within this context?
5. What complexities does reproductive technology bring to definitions of kinship? How is parenthood redefined? Is a woman who carries another couple's child considered the mother also? Why or why not?
6. What is the effect of biotechnology on pregnancy? What ethical issues does it raise?
7. What kind of logic underlies the practice of cloning? Is cloning ethical? Why or why not?

Chapter 12

1. The authors argue that a visit to the doctor is not a neutral event. Comment on this from your own experience.
2. To understand the doctor-patient relationship, we must look at foci of interest, framework of knowledge, and social context. Why are these important? How are these specific aspects illustrated in western biomedicine?
3. What is behavior in illness and how is it socially constructed?
4. What is your individual conception of pain? How does this relate to the cultural construction of pain?
5. What is the formal logic (i.e. the main propositions) upon which biomedicine is based?
6. What do the terms patient compliance and patient non-compliance mean? Why is this significant in relation to the examples presented by the authors?
7. What is the cultural construction of doctors in your specific social setting? In your view does this construction place limitations on processes of healing?

Chapter 13

1. What is Critical Medical Anthropology? What are some of its criticisms? Are they valid? Why or why not?
2. Within the context of CMA, what do the authors mean when they say "there is no such thing as a neutral or value-free social science"? How does this statement shape the way we look at CMA?
3. The authors cite smoking as a coercive habit in which people recognize their actions as free will, but experience an underlying force of coercion. Can you think of any other examples with medical consequences that on the surface appear individualistic but are, in a sense, regulated?
4. Discuss the apparent contradiction that minorities are vulnerable to the coercion of tobacco even though they produce strong resistance to the status quo. Can you give any other examples that correspond to this situation?
5. Cite some examples of indigenous concepts and applications of tobacco. How and why is it utilized? Can you present the "Western" use of tobacco in a ritual context?

Chapter 14

1. The authors conclude that it is feasible to compare different medical systems. What method do they suggest and what uses can be made of it?
2. Can you make any generalizations about the effect that biomedical ideologies have on indigenous systems of medicine? By making generalizations, can you therefore make predictions about the changes that will occur?
3. Is it feasible to separate religion from medical systems? How might this be achieved and can you provide any examples?
4. What is considered collective healing and holistic healing? How do they inter-relate with other aspects of culture (religious, educational)?
5. Is there a clear differentiation between curing and healing? Where are the definitive lines?

References

Chapter 1

Csordas, Thomas J. 1994. *The Sacred Self*. Berkeley: University of California Press.

Fabrega, Horacio, Jr. 1974. *Disease and Social Behavior*. Cambridge, Mass.: MIT Press.

Finkler, Kaja 1994a. *Spiritualist Healers in Mexico: Successes and Failures of Alternative Therapeutics*. South Hadley, Massachusetts: Bergin and Garvey (first published 1985).

Foster, George M. 1994. *Hippocrates' Latin American Legacy*. USA: Gordon and Breach.

Foster, George M. and Barbara Galatin Anderson 1978. *Medical Anthropology*. New York: Alfred Knopf.

Frankel, Stephen 1986. *The Huli Response to Illness*. Cambridge: Cambridge University Press.

Frankel, Stephen and Gilbert Lewis (eds.) 1989. *A Continuing Trial of Treatment: Medical Pluralism in Papua New Guinea*. Boston: Kluwer Academic Publishers.

Geertz, Clifford 1973. Thick description: toward an interpretive theory of culture. *The Interpretation of Cultures*. New York: Basic Books.

Helman, Cecil 1994. *Culture, Health and Illness: An Introduction for Health Professionals*, (3rd ed.). Oxford and Boston: Butterworth-Heinemann.

Kleinman, Arthur 1980. *Patients and Healers in the Context of Culture*. Berkeley: University of California Press.

McElroy, Ann and Patricia K. Townsend 1985. *Medical Anthropology in Ecological Perspective*. Boulder: Westview Press.

Ohnuki-Tierney, Emiko 1984. *Illness and Culture in Contemporary Japan*. Cambridge: Cambridge University Press.

Strathern, Andrew J. 1996. *Body Thoughts*. Ann Arbor: University of Michigan Press.

Chapter 2

Brain, Peter 1986. *Galen on Bloodletting*. Cambridge: Cambridge University Press.

Camporesi, Piero 1995. *Juice of Life: The Symbolic and Magic Significance of Blood*. New York: Continuum.

Colson, A.B. and C. de Armellada 1983. An Amerindian derivation for Latin American Creole illnesses and their treatment. *Social Science and Medicine* 17: 229–248.

Cosminsky, Sheila and Susan Scrimshaw 1980. Medical pluralism on a Guatemala plantation. *Social Science and Medicine* 14B: 267–278.

Crandon-Malamud, L. 1991. *From the Fat of Our Souls: Social Change, Political Process, and Medical Pluralism in Bolivia*. Berkeley: University of California Press.

Escobar, G.J., E. Salazar, and M. Chuy. 1983. Beliefs regarding the etiology and treatment of infantile diarrhea in Lima, Peru. *Social Science and Medicine* 17: 257–269.

Foster, G.M. 1994. *Hippocrates' Latin American Legacy: Humoral Medicine in the New World*. USA: Gordon and Breach.

Foster, George M. and Barbara Galatin Anderson 1978. *Medical Anthropology*. New York: Alfred Knopf.

Furst, Jill 1995. *The Natural History of the Soul in Ancient Mexico*. New Haven: Yale University Press.

Jenkins, Janis and Martha Valiente 1994. Bodily transactions of the passions: *el calor* among El Salvadoran women refugees. In T. Csordas (ed.) *Embodiment and Experience*, pp.163–182. Cambridge: Cambridge University Press.

Kamppinen, M. 1990. Out of balance: Models of the human body in the medico-religious tradition among the Mestizos of the Peruvian Amazon. *Curare* 13(2): 89–97.

Lipp, F.J. 1991. *The Mixe of Oaxaca: Religion, Ritual, and Healing*. Austin: University of Texas Press.

Lloyd, Geoffrey (ed.) 1973. *Hippocratic Writings*. Harmondsworth: Penguin Books.

Lock, Margaret 1980. *East Asian Medicine in Urban Japan: Varieties of Medical Experience*. Berkeley: University of California Press.

Logan, M.H. 1973. Humoral medicine in Guatemala and peasant acceptance of modern medicine. *Human Organization* 32(4): 385–395.

Nutini, Hugo and Jack Roberts 1993. *Blood-Sucking Witchcraft: An Epistemological Study of Anthropomorphic Supernaturalism in Rural Tlaxcala*. Tucson: University of Arizona Press.

Ohnuki-Tierney, Emiko 1984. *Illness and Culture in Contemporary Japan.* Cambridge: Cambridge University Press.

Ortiz de Montellano, B. 1990. *Aztec Medicine, Health, and Nutrition.* New Brunswick: Rutgers University Press.

Pederson, D. and V. Baruffati 1989. Healers, deities, saints, and doctors: elements for the analysis of medical systems. *Social Science and Medicine* 29(4): 487–496.

Scott, J.C. 1990. *Domination and The Arts of Resistance: Hidden Transcripts.* New Haven: Yale University Press.

Trawick, Margaret 1995. Western reflections on Chinese and Indian medicine. In Don Bates (ed.) *Knowledge and the Scholarly Medical Traditions.* Cambridge: Cambridge University Press.

Waxler-Morrison, Nancy E. 1988. Plural medicine in Sri Lanka: Do Ayurvedic and Western medical practices Differ? *Social Science and Medicine* 27(5): 531–544.

Zimmermann, Francis 1982. *The Jungle and the Aroma of Meats: An Ecological Theme in Hindu Medicine.* Berkeley: California University Press.

Chapter 3

Bateson, Gregory 1972. *Steps to an Ecology of Mind.* New York: Ballantine Books.

King, Helen 1998. *Hippocrates' Woman.* London: Routledge.

Strathern, A. 1973. Kinship, descent, and locality: some New Guinea examples. In J.R. Goody (ed.) *The Character of Kinship.* Cambridge: Cambridge University Press.

Strathern, A. and Pamela J. Stewart 1997. The efficacy-entertainment braid revisited: From ritual to commerce in Papua New Guinea. *Journal of Ritual Studies* 11(1): 61–70.

Strathern, A. and Pamela J. Stewart 1998a. Melpa and Nuer ideas of life and death: The rebirth of a comparison. In Lambek, M. and A. Strathern (eds.) *Bodies and Persons: Comparative Perspectives from Africa and Melanesia.* Cambridge: Cambridge University Press, pp. 232–251.

Strathern, A. and Pamela J. Stewart 1998b. Embodiment and communication: Two frames for the analysis of ritual. *Social Anthropology* 6(2):237–251.

Strathern, A. and Pamela J. Stewart 1998c. Seeking personhood: Anthropological accounts and local concepts in Mount Hagen, Papua New Guinea. *Oceania* 68(3): 170–188.

Strathern, A. and Pamela J. Stewart 1999a. Objects, relationships, and meanings: Historical switches in currencies in Mount Hagen, Papua New Guinea. In Joel Robbins and David Akin (eds.) *Money and Modernity: State and Local Currencies in Melanesia.* Association for Social Anthropology in Oceania Monograph Series No. 17. Pittsburgh: University of Pittsburgh Press.

Strathern, A. and Pamela J. Stewart 1999b. *"The Spirit is Coming!" A Photographic-Textual Exposition of the Female Spirit Cult Performance in Mt. Hagen.* Ritual Studies Monograph Series, Monograph No. 1 (forthcoming).

Chapter 4

Brodwin, Paul 1996. *Medicine and Morality in Haiti.* Cambridge: Cambridge University Press.

Finkler, Kaja 1994b. Sacred healing and biomedicine compared. *Medical Anthropology Quarterly* Vol. 8, No. 2, pp. 178–197.

Stewart, Pamela J. and A. Strathern1997a. Sorcery and Sickness: Spatial and Temporal Movements in Papua New Guinea and Australia. Townsville: JCU, *Centre for Pacific Studies Discussion Paper Series* No. 1, pp. 1–27.

Stewart, Pamela J. and A. Strathern (eds.) 1997b. *Millennial Markers.* Townsville: JCU, Center for Pacific Studies.

Stewart, Pamela J. and A. Strathern 1998. Life at the end: Voices and visions from Mt. Hagen, Papua New Guinea. *Zeitschrift für Missionswissenschaft—und Religionswissenschaft,* 4: 227–244.

Chapter 5

Meggitt, M.J. 1957. The Ipili of the Porgera Valley, Western Highlands District, Territory of New Guinea. *Oceania* 28: 31–55.

—— 1973. The Sun and the Shakers: a millenarian cult and its transformations in the New Guinea Highlands. *Oceania* 44(1): 1–37 and 109–126.

Stewart, P.J. 1998. Ritual trackways and sacred paths of fertility. In Jelle Miedema, Cecilia Ode, and Rien Dam (eds.) *Proceedings of the first international interdisciplinary conference, Perspectives on the Bird's Head of Irian Jaya, Indonesia* (Leiden 13–17 1997). Amsterdam: Rodopi, pp. 275–290.

Stewart, P.J. and A. Strathern 1998. Witchcraft, murder and ecological stress: A Duna (Papua New Guinea) case study. *JCU Discussion Papers Series* No. 4.

Stewart, P.J. and A. Strathern n.d.b. Duna songs of sorrow. Sending the spirits away in Papua New Guinea. Ms. in preparation.

Strathern, A. 1996. *Body Thoughts*. Ann Arbor: University of Michigan Press.

Strathern, A.J. and P.J. Stewart 1998. Embodiment and communication: two frames for the analysis of ritual. *Social Anthropology* 6, pt. 2: 237–251.

Strathern, A. and Pamela J. Stewart 1999b. *"The Spirit is Coming!" A Photographic-Textual Exposition of the Female Spirit Cult Performance in Mt. Hagen.* Ritual Studies Monograph Series, Monograph No. 1 (forthcoming).

Telban, Borut 1997. Being and "non-being" in Ambonwari (PNG) ritual. *Oceania* 67: 309–325.

Chapter 6

Ballard, Chris 1994. The Centre Cannot Hold. Trade networks and sacred geography in the Papua New Guinea Highlands. *Archaeology in Oceania* 29(3): 130–148.

Frankel, Stephen 1986. *The Huli Response to Illness*. Cambridge: Cambridge University Press.

Stewart, Pamela J. 1998. Ritual trackways and sacred paths of fertility. In Jelle Miedema, Cecilia Ode, and Rien Dam (eds.) *Proceedings of the first international interdisciplinary conference, Perspectives on the Bird's Head of Irian Jaya, Indonesia* (Leiden 13–17 1997). Amsterdam: Rodopi, pp. 275–290.

Stewart, Pamela J. and Andrew Strathern 1997a. Sorcery and Sickness: Spatial and Temporal Movements in Papua New Guinea and Australia. Townsville: JCU, *Centre for Pacific Studies Discussion Papers Series*, No. 1, pp. 1–27.

Stewart, Pamela J. and Andrew Strathern 1997b. Transecting bisects: Female Spirit cults as a prism of cultural performance in the Hagen, Pangia, and Duna areas of Papua New Guinea. *Okari Research Group Prepublication Working Paper* No. 1, pp. 1–41.

Strathern, Andrew 1977. Souvenirs de folie chez les Wiru. *Journal de la Société des Océanistes* 33: 131–144.

———— 1989. Health care and medical pluralism: cases from Mt. Hagen. In Stephen Frankel and Gilbert Lewis (eds.) *A Continuing Trial of Treatment. Medical Pluralism in Papua New Guinea*. Dordrecht: Kluwer Academic Publishers, pp. 141–154.

Chapter 7

Finkler, Kaja 1994a. *Spiritualist Healers in Mexico*. Massachusetts: Bergin and Garvey (2nd ed., first published 1985).

Chapter 8

Brodwin, Paul 1996. *Medicine and Morality in Haiti: The Contest for Healing Power*. Cambridge: Cambridge University Press.

Cawte, John 1974. *Medicine is the Law: Studies in Psychiatric Anthropology of Australian Tribal Societies*. Honolulu: University of Hawaii Press.

Crandon-Malamud, Libbet 1991. *From the Fat of Our Souls: Social Change, Political Process, and Medical Pluralism in Bolivia*. Berkeley: University of California Press.

Darrouzet, Christopher Patrick 1985. *Sorcery, Salvation, and the Politics of Death in a Lowland New Guinea Society: A Case Study of a Modernizing Culture and Consciousness*. Ph.D. Dissertation. University of North Carolina at Chapel Hill.

Gaines, Attwood D. (ed.) 1992. *Ethnopsychiatry: The Cultural Construction of Professional and Folk Psychiatries*. New York: State University of New York Press.

Janes, Craig R., Ron Stall, and Sandra M. Gifford (eds.) 1986. *Anthropology and Epidemiology*. Dordrecht: D. Reidel.

Pliskin, Karen L. 1987. *Silent Boundaries: Cultural Constraints on Sickness and Diagnosis of Iranians in Israel*. New Haven: Yale University Press.

Read, Janice 1983. *Sorcerers and Healing Spirits: Continuity and Change in an Aboriginal Medical System*. Canberra: Australian National University Press.

Riebe, Inge 1987. Kalam witchcraft: a historical perspective. In Michele Stephen (ed.) *Sorcerer and Witch in Melanesia*. New Brunswick: Rutgers University Press, pp. 211–245.

Stewart, Pamela J. and A. Strathern 1997. Sorcery and Sickness: Spatial and Temporal Movements in Papua New Guinea and Australia. Townsville: JCU, *Centre for Pacific Studies Discussion Papers Series*, No. 1, pp. 1–27.

Strathern, A. 1996. *Body Thoughts*. Ann Arbor: University of Michigan Press.

Warner, W. Lloyd 1969 (1937). *A Black Civilization: A Study of an Australian Tribe*. Gloucester: Peter Smith.

Zelenietz, Marty and Shirley Lindenbaum (eds.) 1981. Sorcery and Social Change in Melanesia. *Social Analysis* 8, spec. issue.

Chapter 9

Blacking, John 1977. Toward an anthropology of the body. In Blacking, J. (ed.) *The Anthropology of the Body*. New York: Academic Press, pp.1–28.

Csordas, Thomas J. 1994 . *The Sacred Self: A Cultural Phenomenology of Charismatic Healing*. Berkeley: University of California Press.

―――― 1997. *Language, Charisma, and Creativity: The Ritual Life of a Religious Community*. Berkeley: University of California Press.

Finkler, Kaja 1985. *Spiritualist Healers in Mexico*. South Hadley, Mass.: Bergin and Garvey. (2nd ed. 1994).

Frank, Jerome and Julia Frank 1993. *Persuasion and Healing*. Baltimore: Johns Hopkins University Press (3rd ed.).

McGuire, Meredith with Debra Kantor 1998. *Ritual Healing in Suburban America*. New Brunswick: Rutgers University Press.

McGuire, Meredith with Debra Kantor 1982. *Pentecostal Catholics: Power, Charisma and Order in a Religious Movement*. Philadelphia: Temple University Press.

Shaara, Lila 1994. *Struggle for Belief; The Expansion of One Religious Community in a Postindustrial Setting*. Ph.D Thesis, University of Pittsburgh.

Strathern, Andrew and Pamela J. Stewart 1998. Seeking personhood. Anthropological accounts and local concepts in Mt. Hagen, New Guinea. *Oceania* 68(3): 170–188.

Chapter 10

Bates, Don (ed.) 1995. *Knowledge and the Scholarly Medical Traditions*. Cambridge: Cambridge University Press.

Bruce-Chwalt, Leonard Jan and Julian de Zulveta 1980. *The Rise and Fall of Malaria in Europe: A Historical-Epidemiological Study*. Oxford University Press, for WHO.

212 · Curing and Healing

Denoon, Donald 1989. *Public Health in Papua New Guinea: Medical Possibility and Social Constraint, 1884–1984*. Cambridge: Cambridge University Press,

Desowitz, Robert S. 1991. *The Malaria Capers: More Tales of Parasites and People, Research and Reality*. New York: W.W. Norton.

Dobson, Mary J. 1997. *Contours of Death and Disease in Early Modern England*. Cambridge: Cambridge University Press.

Hippocrates (Hippocratic Writings) 1978. *Hippocratic Writings* transl. by J. Chadwick and W.N. Mann. (ed.) with an introduction by G.E.R. Lloyd. Harmondsworth: Penguin Books.

Kwiatkowski, Dominic and Kevin Marsh 1997. Development of a malaria vaccine. *The Lancet* 350 (9092): 1696–1701.

Martin, Emily 1994. *Flexible Bodies: Tracking Immunity in American Culture from the Days of Polio to the Age of AIDS*. Boston: Beacon Press.

Miles, John 1997. *Infectious Diseases Colonising the Pacific?* Dunedin; New Zealand: University of Otago Press.

Riebe, Inge 1987. Kalam witchcraft: a in historical perspective. In Michele Stephen (ed.) *Sorcerer and Witch in Melanesia*. New Brunswick: Rutgers University Press, pp. 211–245.

Schuurkamp, Gerrit J.T. 1992. *The Epidemiology of Malaria and Filariasis in the Ok Tedi Region of Western Province, Papua New Guinea*. OTML.

Spencer, Margaret 1994. *Malaria: The Australian Experience 1843–1991*. Townsville: Australian College of Tropical Medicine Publications (James Cook University).

Tanner, Marcel and Carol Vlassoff 1997. Treatment-seeking behavior for malaria: a typology based on endemicity and gender. *Social Science and Medicine* 46(4–5): 523–532.

Wear, Andrew 1995. Epistemology and learned medicine in early modern England. In D. Bates (ed.) *Knowledge and the Scholarly Medical Traditions*. Cambridge University Press, pp.151–174.

Weiss, Brad 1992. Plastic Teeth extraction: the iconography of Haya gastro-sexual affliction. *American Ethnologist* 19(3): 538–552.

Chapter 11

Annas, George J. 1998. The Shadowlands: Secrets, Lies, and Assisted Reproduction. *New England Journal of Medicine* 339: 935–939.

Brady, Ivan (ed.) 1976. *Transactions in Kinship: Adoption and Fosterage in Oceania*. Hawaii: University of Hawaii Press.

Ebin, V. 1994. Interpretations of Infertility: the Aowin People of South-west Ghana. In MacCormack, Carol P. (ed.) *Ethnography of Fertility and Birth*, 2nd edition. Prospect Heights: Waveland Press.

Evans-Pritchard, E.E. 1940. *The Nuer*.Oxford: Oxford University Press.

───── 1951. *Kinship and Marriage among the Nuer*. Oxford: Oxford University Press.

Fox, Robin 1997. *Reproduction and Succession. Studies in Anthropology, Law, and Society*. New Brunswick: Transaction Publishers.

LeRoy, John 1985. *Fabricated World*. Vancouver: University of British Columbia Press.

McGilvray, D.B. 1994. Sexual Power and fertility in Sri Lanka: Batticaloa Tamils and Moors. In MacCormack, Carol P. (ed.) *Ethnography of Fertility and Birth*, 2nd edition. Prospect Heights: Waveland Press.

Meigs, Anna 1989. The cultural construction of reproduction and its relationship to kinship and gender. In Marshall, M. and J.L. Coughey (eds.) *Culture, Kin, and Cognition in Oceania*. Washington, D.C.: American Anthropological Association.

Rapp, Rayna 1993. Accounting for amniocentesis. In Lindenbaum, Shirley and Margaret Lock (eds.) *Knowledge, Power and Practice. The Anthropology of Medicine and Everyday Life*. Berkeley: University of California Press, pp.55–78.

Stewart, Pamela 1998. Ritual trackways and sacred paths of fertility. In Jelle Miedema, Cecilia Ode, and Rien Dam (eds.) *Proceedings of the first international interdisciplinary conference, Perspectiveson the Bird's Head of Irian Jaya, Indonesia* (Leiden 13–17 Oct. 1997). Amsterdam: Rodopi, pp. 275–290.

Stewart, P. and A. Strathern 1998. Netbags Revisited: Cultural Narratives from Papua New Guinea. *Pacific Studies* Vol. 20, No. 2, pp.1–30

Strathern, Andrew 1973. Kinship, descent, and locality: Some New Guinea examples. In Goody, J.R. (ed.) *The Character of Kinship*. Cambridge: Cambridge University Press.

───── 1977. *Myths and Legends from Mt. Hagen*. (Trans. of Vicedom 1943–8 vol. 3). Port Moresby: Institute of PNG Studies.

Strathern, A. and Pamela J. Stewart 1998a. Embodiment and Communication: Two frames for the analysis of ritual. *Social Anthropology* 6(2): 231–251.

Strathern, A. and Pamela J. Stewart 1998b. Melpa and Nuer ideas of life and death: The rebirth of a comparison. In Lambek, M. and A.J. Strathern (eds.) *Bodies and Persons: Comparative Perspectives from Africa and Melanesia*. Cambridge: Cambridge University Press, pp. 232–251.

Strauss, Hermann and H. Tischner 1962. *Die Mi-Kultur der Hagenberg-Stämme*. Hamburg: Cram, de Gruyter and Co.
Vicedom,Georg F. and H. Tischner 1943–8. *Die Mbowamb* (3 vols.) Vol. 3 *Mythen und Erzählungen*. Hamburg: Friederichsen, de Gruyter and Co.

Chapter 12

Bourhis, R.Y., et al. 1989. Communication in the hospital setting: A survey of medical and everyday language use amongst patients, nurses and doctors. *Social Science and Medicine* 28(4): 339–346.
Cicourel, A.V. 1992. The interpenetration of communicative contexts: examples from medical encounters. In A. Duranti and C. Goodwin (eds.) *Rethinking Context*. Cambridge: Cambridge University Press, pp. 291–310.
Finkler, Kaja 1991. *Physicians at Work, Patients in Pain*. Boulder: Westview Press
——— 1994c. *Women in Pain: Gender and Morbidity in Mexico*. Philadelphia: University of Pennsylvania Press.
Frankenberg, Ronald (ed.) 1992. *Time, Health and Medicine*. London: Sage Publications.
Good, Mary-Jo Delvecchio, Paul E. Brodwin, Byron J. Good, and Arthur Kleinman (eds.) 1992. *Pain in Human Experience*. Berkeley: University of California Press.
Good, Byron (1994) *Medicine, Rationality, and Experience: An Anthropological Perspective*, Cambridge: Cambridge University Press.
Gunnarrson, B.-L., Per Linell, and Bengt Nordberg (eds.) 1995. *The Construction of Professional Discourse*. London: Longman.
Hahn, Robert A. 1985. A world of internal medicine: Portrait of an internist. In R. Hahn and A. Gaines (eds.) *Physicians of Western Medicine. Anthropological Approaches to Theory and Practice*. Dordrecht: D. Reidel Publishing Company, pp. 51–114.
Helman, Cecil 1994. *Culture, Health and Illness*. Boston: Butterworth-Heinemann.
Higgs, J. and Jones, M. (eds.) 1995. *Clinical Reasoning in the Health Professions*. Boston: Butterworth-Heinemann.
Julian, D.G., K.I. Lie, and L. Wilhelmsen (eds.) 1982. *What is Angina?* Molndal (Sweden): A.B. Hassle.
Katz, Pearl 1985. How surgeons make decisions. In R. Hahn and A. Gaines (eds.) *Physicians of Western Medicine*. Dordrecht: D. Reidel, pp. 155–176.
Laine, Christine and Frank Davidoff 1996. Patient-centered medicine: A professional evolution. *Journal of the American Medical Association* 275(2): 152–156.

Legato, M. J. and C. Colman 1991. *The Female Heart*. New York: Simon and Schuster.

Lewis, Gilbert 1993. Some studies of social causes of and cultural response to disease. In C.G.N. Mascie-Taylor (ed.) *The Anthropology of Disease*. Oxford: Oxford University Press, pp. 73–124.

Lock, M. and Gordon D. (eds.) 1988. *Biomedicine Examined*. Dordrecht: Kluwer Academic Publishers.

Maretzki, Thomas W. 1985. Including the physician in healer-centered research: Retrospect and prospect. In R. Hahn and A. Gaines (eds.) *Physicians of Western Medicine*. Dordrecht: D. Reidel, pp. 23–50.

——— 1989. Cultural Variations in Biomedicine. The *Kur* in West Germany. *Medical Anthropology Quarterly* 3(1): 23–50.

Medical Anthropology Quarterly 12(3) 1998. Papers on clinical decision-making by Linda M. Hunt, Cheryl Mattingley and Linda C. Garro.

Mischler, E. 1986a. *The Discourse of Medicine: Dialectics of Medical Interviews*. Norwood, NJ:ABLEX.

Novack, Dennis H., Suchman, Anthony L., Clark, William, Epotesh, Ronald M., Najberg, Eva, and Kaplan, Craig 1997. Calibrating the physician: personal awareness and effective patient care. *Journal of the American Medical Association* 278(6): 502–509.

Pantano, J.A. 1990. *Living with Angina*. New York: Harper & Row.

Roter, Debra L., Stewart, Moira, Putnam, Samuel M., Lipkin, Mack, Jr., Stiles, William, and Ijui, Thomas S. 1987. Communication patterns of primary care physicians. *Journal of the American Medical Association* 277(4): 350–356

Singer, Merrill 1987. Cure, care and control: an ectopic encounter with biomedical obstetrics. In Hans A. Baer (ed.) *Encounters with Biomedicine: Case Studies in Medical Anthropology*. New York: Gordon and Breach Publishers, pp. 248–268.

Stewart, Pamela J. and A. Strathern 1997. Doctor to doctor: Health care practitioner perspectives on Diabetes Mellitus. Paper presented at the Session, "Diabetes Care and the Dynamics of Power Relations" at the Society for Applied Anthropology conference in Seattle, Washington in 1997.

Strathern, A.J. 1996. *Body Thoughts*. Ann Arbor: University of Michigan Press.

Tanner, C. 1993. Rethinking clinical judgement. In N. Diekelmann and M. Rather (eds.) *Transforming RN Education: Dialogue and Debate*. New York: N.L.N. Press.

Waitzkin, H. 1991. *The Politics of Medical Encounters. How Patients and Doctors Deal with Social Problems*. New Haven:Yale University Press.

Chapter 13

Baer, Hans A., Merrill Singer, and Ida Susser 1997. *Medical Anthropology and the World System: A Critical Perspective*. Westport: Bergin and Garvey.

Knauft, Bruce B. 1996. *Genealogies for the Present in Cultural Anthropology*. London and New York: Routledge.

Kroeber, Alfred 1939. Cultural elements and distribution xv: Salt, dogs, and tobacco. *Anthropological Records* 6(1).

Larkin, Philip 1988. *Collected Poems*. Edited by Anthony Thwaite. London: Marvell Press.

Marcus, George and Michael Fischer 1986. *Anthropology as Cultural Critique*. Chicago: University of Chicago Press.

Marshall, Mac 1979. Introduction. In M. Marshall (ed.) *Beliefs, Behaviors and Alcoholic Beverages*. Ann Arbor: University of Michigan Press, pp. 2–11.

McElroy, Ann. 1996. Should medical anthropology be political? *Medical Anthropology Quarterly* 10(4): 519–522.

Press, Irwin 1990. Levels of explanation and cautions for a critical clinical anthropology. *Social Science and Medicine* Vol. 30., No. 9, pp. 1001–1009.

Strathern, Andrew 1993. *Landmarks*. Ohio: Kent State University Press.

Wilpert, Johannes 1987. *Tobacco and Shamanism in South America*. New Haven: Yale University Press.

Chapter 14

Brody, Howard 1992. *The Healer's Power*. New Haven: Yale University Press.

Danforth, Loring M. 1989. *Firewalking and Religious Healing: The Anasteria of Greece and the American Firewalking Movement*. Princeton: Princeton University Press.

Finkler, Kaja 1994b. Sacred healing and biomedicine compared. *Medical Anthropology Quarterly* 8(2): 178–197.

Gevitz, Norman (ed.) 1988. *Other Healers: Unorthodox Medicine in America*. Baltimore: John Hopkins University Press.

Good, Byron J. 1994. *Medicine, Rationality and Experience*. Cambridge: Cambridge University Press.

Kleinman, Arthur 1988. *Rethinking Psychiatry: From Cultural Category to Personal Experience*. New York: The Free Press.

Lindenbaum, Shirley and Margaret Lock (eds.) 1993. *Knowledge, Power and Practice: The Anthropology of Medicine in Everyday Life.* Berkeley: University of California Press.

Lock, Margaret and Deborah Gordon 1988. *Biomedicine Examined.* Dordrecht: Kluwer Publishers.

McClain, Carol Shepherd (ed.) 1989. *Women as Healers: Cross-Cultural Perspectives.* New Brunswick: Rutgers University Press.

Parker, Arthur C. 1909. Secret medicine societies of the Seneca. *American Anthropologist*, N.S., Vol. XI, No. 2. (April-June): pp. 161–185.

Vogel, Virgil J. 1970. *American Indian Medicine.* Norman: University of Oklahoma Press.

Index